ELDER PRACTICE

SOCIAL PROBLEMS AND SOCIAL ISSUES

Leon Ginsberg, Editor

ELDER PRACTICE

A MULTIDISICIPLINARY APPROACH TO WORKING WITH OLDER ADULTS IN THE COMMUNITY

Terry Tirrito
Ilene Nathanson
Nieli Langer

UNIVERSITY OF SOUTH CAROLINA PRESS

Copyright © 1996 University of South Carolina

Published in Columbia, South Carolina, by the
University of South Carolina Press

Manufactured in the United States of America

00 99 98 97 96 5 4 3 2 1

Tirrito, Terry, 1945–
    Elder practice: a multidisciplinary approach to working with
older adults in the community/by Terry Tirrito, Ilene Nathanson,
and Nieli Langer.
        p.   cm.—(Social problems and social issues)
    Includes bibliographical references and index.
    ISBN 1–57003–075–8 (pbk.)
    1. Aged—Services for—United States. 2. Aged—Care—United
States. 3. Community health services for the aged—United States.
I. Nathanson, Ilene. II. Langer, Nieli. III. Title. IV. Series.
HV1461.T57 1996
362.6'0973—dc20   95–32516

To my husband, Sal, for his patience and support. To my mother, Anna Terrasi, whose life and death inspired this book. To Leon Ginsberg without whose encouragement this book would not have been written.

Terry Tirrito

I wish to acknowledge the editorial contributions of two dear friends and colleagues, Cynthia Wagner, M.S.W., and Jennifer Fowler, J.D., who personify the spirit of collaboration.

Ilene Nathanson

To the other four Langers: Oded, Erris, Orli, and Chemie who give special meaning to the term *familial support.*

Nieli Langer

CONTENTS

Editor's Preface   ix

Introduction   1

1. The Scope of the Issue:
    The Need for a Multidisciplinary Approach   6

2. A Multidisciplinary Approach:
    Impact on the Need for Services   23

3. Health Issues:
    Impact on the Need for Services   37

4. Mental Health Issues:
    Impact on the Need for Services   52

5. Legal Dilemmas:
    Implications for Health and Social Functioning   66

6. Religiosity, Spirituality, and Ethical Issues:
    Including Religious Organizations in the Service Network   79

7. Cultural Competency:
    The Impact of Ethnicity on the Need for Services   95

8. Social Functioning:
    Assessment and Impact on the Need for Services   115

9. The Role of Community Practitioners:
    The Service Network   140

10. Elder Assessment:
    A Multidisciplinary Approach   152

11. The Coordination of a Referral and Treatment Plan   174

12. Implicatons of the Multidisciplinary Approach   187

Conclusion   193
Appendix: Multidisciplinary Screening Instrument (MSI)   196
Index   199

EDITOR'S PREFACE

Social and individual problems are increasingly a concern of United States society. As the nation has become more heavily industrialized, metropolitan, and complex in other ways, the severity and magnitude of human need become larger priorities for the society as a whole. In an earlier time and in rural, agrarian societies, families were better able to cope, without the help of others, with family members who had mental illnesses and developmental disabilities such as mental retardation. Older family members could be cared for within the family. Those who committed crimes or were otherwise abusive could be disciplined by the family or, in extreme cases, the village.

In industrial, metropolitan societies such as the one we have in the United States, families are nuclear—consisting only of parents and their children—rather than the extended families of the past in which aunts, uncles, cousins, grandparents, and others were a part. Out of the major changes in living have emerged the human services professions, including counseling, rehabilitation, social work, and many others.

The members of these professions, one of the primary audiences to whom this series, Social problems and Issues, is directed, play a constantly growing role in United States society through their application of human programs and services. The series is designed, in large part, to help students of the human services as well as established practitioners remain knowledgeable about current developments and thinking in these fields of endeavor. Another audience for this series, perhaps the second most important, are those who use the human services and their families. Consumers need to understand the underlying ideas of the human services professionals and the methods they use in addressing problems.

This work, by Terry Tirrito, Ilene Nathanson, and Nieli Langer, all three of whom are accomplished scholars and practitioners with older people, is an imaginative look at some modern approaches to working with older adults and their families. At the time this book was completed, some 13 percent of the U.S.

population was 65 or older, and nearly half that group, 8.4 percent, was over 75. More of the human services efforts and expenditures in the U.S. are devoted to older people than to any other group, a proportion that is likely to expand as the total population becomes older. The numbers alone make this book, which is an excellent example of modern, practical thinking about services for the aging, an important addition to this series. It is a pleasure to add this fine piece of scholarship to the volumes of Social Problems and Social Issues.

—Leon Ginsberg

ELDER PRACTICE

INTRODUCTION

History is a cyclical process. Discussions of fashion trends or developments in health care reveal its repetitive nature. Everyone over the age of forty can easily recall that fashion blight of the 1960s, bell-bottom pants. Are they as quick to recall the War on Poverty and efforts of the Kennedy and Johnson Administrations to fill gaps in service delivery through the inauguration of such landmark legislation as Medicare, Medicaid, and the neighborhood health centers? Bell-bottoms are back, and so is the concern with universal health coverage. Although the rhetoric has changed and the proposed solutions to gaps in health delivery have been altered by an increasing concern with cost control, the real answers to solving our "health crisis" lie in solutions that are timeless and basic.

Any organizational system is only as effective as the individuals involved choose to make it. We can change health financing mechanisms, and we can ration care. We can increase the use of sanctions in efforts to maintain quality. We can emphasize primary care over more acute treatment modalities. We cannot, however, force practitioners to want to work together for the benefit of their clients and patients. The desire to help must come from an internal sense of responsibility and commitment to a standard of mutual cooperation. The need for helping is timeless.

Many respected health care analysts (Freidson 1975) have argued for preserving the discretion of practitioners in controlling their work. Professional discretion is viewed as paramount to the skillful delivery of services and a critical part of the professional's sense of responsibility.

The basic questions that must be answered to promote real quality care, and which are the emphasis of this book, are: How does one encourage cooperation among practitioners, and, having done so, how does one establish the opportunity for more skillful coordination of services?

The purpose of this book is to develop and explain a multidisciplinary approach to working with older adults in areas related to health, legal, financial, and social functioning. There has been a dramatic increase in the population of older adults. National data documenting this increase have generated a great deal of interest in planning services and programs for older Americans. There are thirty-one million people over the age of sixty five years and three million over the age of eighty-five years who will require the attention of professionals in various disciplines.

With more of the elderly being served in the community, there is a need to translate institutional norms of interdisciplinary practice into a model of community-based practice. The problem of providing community services to a rapidly growing elderly population is a central issue to policy makers and human service providers. A key issue of the Clinton presidential election was excessive expenditures and gaps in health services delivery. While legislative officials are seeking solutions to problems of financing and ensuring quality health care, professional practitioners must come to grips with the complications of managing the chronic care needs of older people.

Chronic care requires different treatment strategies than acute care. Many older people suffer from chronic medical conditions, such as arthritis, diabetes, hypertension, heart disease, and visual and hearing impairments. In addition, problems in social functioning, resulting from physical and social losses related to old age—for example, retirement or widowhood—may directly impact upon an individual's medical or psychological health. Older people can easily be caught in a negative spiral of frailty in which social, medical, and mental health problems become inexorably intertwined. The multidisciplinary approach outlined in this book is designed to offset these difficulties. Preventive intervention requires that each professional person understand the scope of the health, social, and legal conditions impacting the older person and make appropriate referrals to other professionals for solutions.

Two principal objectives of this book are to enable professional practitioners and students in each discipline to make comprehensive assessments of the range of service needs of their older adult clients; to enable professional practitioners and students, in each discipline, to make appropriate referrals, and to establish linkages with other disciplines providing services to older adults in the community. A model for screening, assessing, and implementing a treatment plan for the older adult client is presented with an emphasis on describing the functions of various practitioners. We will present in this book a comprehensive assessment instrument, the Multidisciplinary Screening Instrument (MSI), for use by the various disciplines.

This book attempts to fill a gap that has existed in the gerontology literature. Our frame of reference is community-based practice. The interaction of various professionals in the life of a community's older adults has been ignored. Until this time the focus of scholarship has been on nursing care, on case management, and on ensuring access of older adults to formal services. It is vital that those in private practice in various fields such as psychiatry, law, nutrition, finance, recreation, and religion become involved with the traditional helping disciplines of medicine, nursing, and social work. It is hoped that this book will be used by practicing professionals in a variety of health-related disciplines. Graduate programs in social work, law, medicine, nursing, and psychology can find this book useful in providing students with a perspective that emphasizes an integrated community practice.

The book represents a mixture of theoretical concepts and concrete applications. Chapter 1 discusses the scope of the issue. It describes the demographics of the older population living in institutions and those living in the community. The costs of institutional care and the costs of community care are presented, including a discussion of Medicare and Medicaid. Finally, the bias in our society toward institutionalization and the current trend toward the development of a multidisciplinary approach toward community care are examined.

Chapter 2 examines the multidisciplinary approach in general. Multidisciplinary activity is defined, and a review of the literature looks at multidisciplinary approaches in selected disciplines such as nursing, medicine, and public health. The problems encountered in multidisciplinary activity are examined, and the team approach in nursing homes and hospitals is presented. Finally, community-based practice is discussed, and knowledge necessary for the community practitioner is offered.

Chapter 3 discusses health issues such as the differences between normal and pathological aging. The need for a practitioner to be knowledgeable about the impact of health issues upon older adults and the relationship of health problems in the screening of psychosocial problems is explained. Data are presented on the prevalence of the most common diseases and of functional problems such as mobility, visual and hearing problems, incontinence, and intestinal problems.

Chapter 4 examines mental health issues. The authors examine the identification and prevalence of mental health problems and the current methods for treatment, including psychotherapeutic interventions. Organic and functional mental disorders that commonly affect older adults—such as cognitive disorders, schizophrenia, paranoia, depression, and anxiety—are examined. The prevalence, identification, and treatment of Alzheimer's disease and related dementias are described. Finally, commonly used psychotropic medications are discussed.

Chapter 5 examines the legal and financial dilemmas that typically confront older people, such as retirement, estate planning, and planning for incapacity. The implications of financial and legal issues in the screening of underlying psychosocial problems are discussed, and connections are made between legal and health problems, and especially mental health problems.

Chapter 6 presents ethical and spiritual issues. The influence of religion upon the well-being of older adults has been noted in the literature and will be discussed in this chapter. Religious institutions and religious leaders are being challenged to provide programs and services for the increasing numbers of older adults in their congregations.

Chapter 7 examines cultural competency and asks the question: How does one become a culturally competent practitioner? Chapter 8 examines social functioning to determine who are the vulnerable elderly and how their connections to relevant service systems can be improved.

Chapter 9 presents the community practitioners. Geriatrician, geropsychiatrists, geropsychotherapists, social workers, geriatric nurses, geriatric case managers, geriatric nutritionists, geriatric financial advisors, and religious leaders are some of the professional practitioners who serve older adults in the community. The authors discuss their specific roles in helping older adults and how each of these practitioners can become a source of referral and treatment.

Chapter 10 presents the Multidisciplinary Screening Instrument (MSI). The MSI was developed to assess and to screen older clients for appropriate referral and treatment by community practitioners. This chapter illustrates how the MSI is used.

Chapter 11 presents the coordination of the referral and treatment plan. Chapter 12 discusses the implications for the use of this model in multidisciplinary community practice. The implications for training, service delivery, education, research, and policy development are presented by the authors.

Perhaps the book's greatest contributions lie in its emphasis on the multidisciplinary process and in its ultimate focus on the individuals behind the professional roles and functions. The book winds its way back to a consideration of that timeless and basic component of quality care, the professional service provider. What can be done to foster mutual cooperation among professionals who are accustomed to operating independently of one another's influence? This is the crucial question addressed in this book. It reflects its ideological foundation: the assumption that organizational systems are only as good as people choose to make them.

The case material that is included in the book represents composite experiences and is designed to highlight principles for screening and assessment and for conflict resolution among practitioners.

Finally, the book includes a discussion of the implications of the multidisciplinary approach for policy and education. The book's primary target of concern is the professional practitioner. We recognize, however, that policy and education impact service delivery; thus, we address these influences upon professional behavior.

REFERENCE

Freidson, E. (1975). *Doctoring together: A study of professional social control.* Chicago: University of Chicago Press.

Chapter 1

THE SCOPE OF THE ISSUE
The Need for a Multidisciplinary Approach

The increase in the population of older adults, especially the "old-old," is having a significant impact upon the services that professionals provide for this group of people. This book is written to aid community professional practitioners. The authors realize that, although many books have been written for case managers, books have not been available which address the multidisciplinary activity of community professional practitioners. The community practitioner frequently works alone with his or her clients, having little or no contact with other professionals. It is the intent of this book to provide a framework for community practitioners to increase their collaborative activity and to provide effective and efficient services to improve the quality of life of older adults. To find help in the community, an older adult frequently must seek the assistance of many professionals from a range of disciplines.

The physician is generally the primary provider of health and medical services. The physician frequently comes into contact with older adults with multiple problems and is often a primary source of referral to other professionals. The lawyer is usually the principal person who advises the older client about legal issues relating to finances, wills, estate planning, and the transfer of funds. The social worker may encounter a client who is referred by an agency or hospital and must be linked to social services or mental health services. The nurse is usually referred by a physician to monitor nursing procedures in the home. Nurses are usually not solo practitioners and are affiliated with a private or public agency. A spiritual leader may become involved when families are seeking solace from the multiple stresses of caregiving, morbidity, or pending mortality. Mental health professionals are found in mental health clinics and in private practice. Studies suggest that older adults do not utilize services from community mental health clinics as frequently as other groups (Turner 1993).

Therefore, the older adult who is experiencing mental health problems such as anxiety or depression may seek treatment with a geriatric psychiatrist or geriatric psychotherapist in the local community. Transportation difficulties hinder seeking treatment in another community or a nearby major city.

What has been missing in these treatment activities is the collaboration of community professionals. How can they coordinate their activities in the best interests of the client? How can they accurately assess the client's needs? How can they refer the client to the appropriate professional for services? In most cases an older adult has not been appropriately referred and treated by community professionals because of the lack of coordinated and collaborative activity in the community.

POPULATION PROJECTIONS

In 1990 the average life expectancy was 78.8 years for females and 71.9 years for males. Women who are age 65 can expect to live an additional 18.6 years, while men can expect to live an additional 14.3 years (Grant and Johnson 1985). It is reported that about four out of five individuals can expect to reach age 80 (Hooyman and Kiyak 1993). Additionally, 88 percent of those 65 years old will celebrate their seventieth birthday, and 82 percent of those 70 years old will reach 75 years of age (Grant and Johnson 1985).

Projections for the future suggest that life expectancy at birth is expected to increase from the current 74.9 years to 77.6 years in 2005 and to 81.2 in 2080 (Hooyman and Kiyak 1993). Females born in 2005 are expected to reach age 81 years; males in that birth cohort will reach age 74. Of particular interest to health planners is the changing proportion of those over 75 years of age, due to their more frequent use of health and social services. These predictions do not take into account new diseases that could increase the mortality risks for men and women. For example, if AIDS continues to be a fatal disease that infects younger males more than females, it could change the ratio of males to females surviving to old age. Death rates by heart disease and hypertension have already begun to decline, however, and may narrow the sex differential and increase life expectancy even more.

Most of the gains have occurred in the early years of life because of the eradication of many diseases that caused high infant and childhood mortality. In addition, we have had significant increases in survival beyond age sixty-five due to advances in medicine and technology. A hundred years ago adults died from acute diseases such as influenza and pneumonia. Today, and in the future, survival from these diseases will create a need for more care for chronic and long-term conditions. The result is a growing number of people who are surviv-

7

ing to old age. The percentage of those over sixty-five years has increased by 22.3 percent from 1980 to 1990 (Ginsberg 1992).

The Oldest-Old

The population aged eighty-five and older is referred to as the "oldest-old" (Hooyman and Kiyak 1993). This group has grown more rapidly than any other age group in our country. In 1990, of the thirty-one million persons age sixty-five and over in the United States, 32 percent were seventy-five to eighty-four years old, while another 10 percent were age eighty-five and over. Those over eighty-five have increased by 300 percent from 1960 to 1990. The number of eighty-five and over was 3,080,000 in 1990 (Ginsberg 1992). Their numbers are expected to reach 4.6 million in the year 2000 and 8 million in 2030. This tremendous growth will take place before the "baby boomers" reach old age, because this latter group will begin to turn eighty-five about 2030. Baby boomers usually refers to those born between 1946 and 1964. The impact of such a surge of older Americans will be dramatic. Projections by the U.S. Census Bureau also suggest a substantial increase in the population age one hundred or older. In 1989 it was estimated that 61,000 Americans were one hundred or older. These numbers are expected to increase to 100,000 by the year 2000 and to 363,000 by 2030. This group can be expected to place increased demands on many social systems in our country, including housing, health care, economic, and social services.

Also, in 1989, ninety-five percent of the population over sixty-five years of age lived in the community, while 5 percent were institutionalized (Gutheil 1990). Older adults living in the community generally function independently, with minimal assistance, among those age sixty-five to seventy-five. Those age seventy-five to eighty-five indicate having more problems in carrying out daily activities and tend to be more frail physically. Americans over eighty-five years of age are most impaired in performing the "activities of daily living" (ADL). Some persons are described as "at risk" and will need institutionalization. Women are at greater risk because they live longer than men and are thus more likely to be living alone, and they have higher rates of chronic illnesses. Social vulnerability combined with multiple chronic conditions prevent independent functioning by the elderly and contribute to risk for institutionalization (Grant and Johnson 1985). The World Health Organization defines *disability* as impairment in the ability to complete multiple daily tasks. It is estimated that more than 20 percent of older adults have a mild degree of disability in their daily activities. Only 4 percent are severely disabled. It is indicated that disabilities and the need for assistance increase with age. About 46 percent of those over eighty-five years old are disabled, as compared to about 13 percent of those age sixty-five to seventy-four and 25 percent of those age seventy-five to eighty-four (Hooyman and Kiyak 1993). Hooyman reports that, in 1987, 5.2 million persons sixty-five or older needed assistance in order to remain in the community, and this figure is projected to be 7.2 million by the year 2000, 10.1 million by 2020, and 14.4 million by 2050.

Who are the oldest-old? Generally, women dominate this group. Seventy percent of Americans eighty-five years old and older are women. Educational level in this group is lower than for those age sixty-five to seventy-four (8.6 years versus 12.2), and most are widowed, divorced, or have never been married (77.2 percent vs. 62 percent). Older women are less well-off financially than are older men (Ginsberg 1992). Women are more likely to have multiple health problems that result in physical frailty, and up to 50 percent may have some form of cognitive impairment. The number of impairments and chronic illnesses rises with age. Almost 25 percent of the oldest-old live in institutional settings (nursing homes, groups homes, or hospitals). More than half the population in nursing homes are reported to be the oldest-old. It is estimated, however, that for every nursing home resident there are three people of equal functioning who are living in the community (Harrington, Newcomer, and Estes 1985).

Frailty versus Well-Being

This picture of a dramatic growth in the number of frail older adults suggests changing care patterns for the future. The need for institutionalization appears to remain constant. Increasing emphasis on community care is essential, however, if we are to manage with scarce resources and provide older adults with adequate care.

Whether to build more institutions or expand community services continues to be debated. An argument has been put forth by Fries (1980) suggesting that, in future years, more people will achieve the maximum life span because of healthier lifestyles during their earlier years. Fries argues that future cohorts will have fewer debilitating illnesses and will, in fact, experience "compressed morbidity," which suggests only a few years of major illness in very old age and then death. If this process occurs, it will have a significant impact on social and health services needed by future generations: if older adults are healthier, they will not need increased medical services but will, instead, demand more employment services and leisure activities.

Other researchers have analyzed results of the National Health Interview Survey and put forth different predictions. Verbrugge (1985), analyzing cohorts from 1958 to 1985, noted that cohorts of middle-aged and older persons reported more short-term disability than did previous cohorts. Morbidity rates increased during this twenty-seven-year period for major life-threatening diseases (e.g., heart disease, cancer, diabetes, and hypertension) as well as for non-life-threatening diseases (e.g., arthritis and osteoporosis), but mortality rates did not increase. Verbrugge concludes that, although medical technology has prevented death from some acute conditions, older people are experiencing more chronic conditions than before. Chronic conditions will require some type of care, and certain conditions will necessitate institutional care. Yet a shift in previously held attitudes can mean that much of the treatment that has traditionally been provided in hospitals or nursing homes will be offered in the community, which is said to be the preferred choice of older adults (Cox 1990).

Others have suggested that the average period of diminished activity will increase because of the growing number of old people who are likely to have multiple chronic illnesses and because some diseases are likely to begin in old age (Schneider and Brody 1983). Preventive health care is being studied to examine how prevention can prolong the healthy period of old age and delay the onset of frailty (Johnson and Wolinsky 1994). Health status is said to involve the interplay of physical, social, and psychological factors. Environmental factors are some of the most significant factors affecting health status. Health risk factor analysis indicates that variations in health-related behaviors and lifestyles are affected by environmental factors (Johnson and Wolinsky 1994).

The concept of "active versus dependent life expectancy" (Katz et al. 1983) distinguishes between merely living a long life and living a healthy life into old age. Debate continues on what constitutes the quality of life for older adults. Policy makers have not yet resolved the issue and continue to promote institutional care and the medical model. There is overwhelming evidence that home care is the preference of most older adults (Cox 1990). The United States government has suggested plans for the improvement of community-based care. It seems, however, that a major source of impetus for this movement must come from older Americans themselves if these policies are to be enacted.

Rates of Institutionalization

The vast majority of older persons do not live in institutions such as nursing homes, boardinghouses, and psychiatric hospitals; only 5 percent of them do. Yet approximately 25 percent of all people over age sixty-five will spend time in a nursing home at some point in later life (Gutheil 1990). Estimates of a person's risk of admission to a nursing home are as high as 50 percent, ranging from 30 percent for men to 50 percent for women (Hooyman and Kiyak 1993). Each year more than a million older persons leave long-term care institutions, with the numbers evenly divided, regarding their reasons for leaving, among returning home, transferring to other facilities, and death (National Center for Health Statistics [NCHS] 1986).

The United States has lower rates of institutionalization than other developed countries. The smallest proportion is Germany (about 4 percent); the highest are Canada (8.7 percent), Sweden (8.7 percent to 10.5 percent), and Switzerland (9 percent). In some countries, such as Greece, Turkey, and Argentina, less than 1 percent of older adults are in long-term care facilities (Hooyman and Kiyak 1993). In other countries, including Japan and Germany, hospitals provide both long-term care and acute care, so the total number of institutionalized elderly is much higher there.

It is expected that the number of older persons in nursing homes will increase in the United States as the population of the oldest-old increases. It has been estimated that this increase will be by 58 percent from 1978 to 2003 if constant mortality rates are assumed and by more than 115 percent if mortality rates decline (NCHS 1989). The average age of nursing home residents is eighty-two, and women are disproportionately represented. The number of all persons aged sixty-five to seventy-four represents 1.2 percent of all persons in nursing homes. This figure increases to 23 percent among those who are aged eighty-five and above. The primary factors that indicate at-risk populations for institutionalization are age (those eighty-five and older), having recently been admitted to a hospital, living in retirement housing rather than being a homeowner, having no spouse at home, having some degree of cognitive impairment, and having one or more problems with the instrumental activities of daily living. In one study these risk factors, in combination, indicated a 62 percent chance of institutionalization within thirty months and a 75 percent chance within seven years (Hooyman and Kiyak 1993).

Nursing Homes

Nursing homes are relatively new living arrangements. Few nursing homes existed prior to the late 1930s and early 1940s. The enactment of Medicare and Medicaid in 1965 gave the impetus for the development of nursing homes. From 1963 to 1973 the number of nursing home beds doubled (Grant and Johnson 1985). Throughout our country's history, poverty and other social problems, such as mental illness, were managed by institutionalization. Prior to 1935, and the Social Security Act, older Americans who were poor lived in almshouses

11

and boardinghouses. After 1965 nursing homes became the solution for providing care to the chronically ill, the mentally ill, the homeless, and the poor. The long-term care institution as it is known today developed in the 1960s. Patients with chronic illnesses were transferred from acute care hospitals to nursing homes, which were influenced by the medical model of care practiced in these acute care settings. In the 1970s the deinstitutionalization of patients in mental hospitals added a new population to nursing homes. The growth of the nursing home industry has also been affected by changing trends in our society, such as declining family size, growth in the population of older adults, and an increase in the numbers of employed women, who were traditionally family caregivers.

The nursing home has become home to the poor, the disabled, individuals with chronic illnesses, and persons with mental illness. The nursing home is unable to meet the goals and objectives society has assigned to it. Critics of nursing homes trace many difficulties to reliance on the medical model of care. The organization of the nursing home is based on the organizational structure of a hospital, and health problems are the main concern of the staff. Psychological and social needs are considered only to the extent that they affect the outcome of an acute illness (Johnson and Grant 1985). The assessment of a disease is made by a professional staff, whose focus is on pathology.

The nursing home, as an all purpose solution to the health problems of the elderly, has created a set of iatrogenic problems; increased dependency, depression and social isolation among the aged. In the United States, although not in many European nations, institutional care of the elderly is conceived and financed as a health service even though institutional placement provides a complete social context for an individual and obviously constitutes a rather dramatic intervention. (Johnson and Grant 1985, 142)

Nursing Home Residents

Institutionalization is not used solely to treat medical problems. A majority of nursing home residents are functionally impaired and are unable to live independently in the community. A primary reason for the institutionalization of older adults is the absence of a caregiver or social support network. Up to 25 percent of nursing home placements are precipitated by a caregiver's illness or death. In 1985, 80 percent of the nursing home population was without a spouse; the majority were widowed. Over 90 percent of nursing home residents are white, compared to 7 percent who are African American, 2.5 percent who are Hispanic, and less than 0.5 percent who are Native American or Asian American. The underrepresentation of ethnic minority groups appears to reflect cultural differences in the willingness to institutionalize, the availability of family supports, and the availability of long-term care facilities. In one study these risk factors, in combination, indicated a 62 percent chance of institutionalization within thirty months and a 75 percent chance within seven years. The cognitively impaired elderly reportedly constitute from 50 to 70 percent of the nursing home population. The projected increase in the incidence of Alzheimer's disease, from four million to eight million Americans in the year 2000, will add significantly to the number of older persons in nursing homes. Although not a part of normal aging, the likelihood of experiencing dementia does increase with advancing age. As more people live to be over seventy years of age, the number of persons with dementia is expected to increase, between 1980 and 2005, by 44 percent among whites and 72 percent among African Americans. This difference in rate of dementia between African Americans and whites is attributed to increased longevity among African Americans. The most common irreversible dementia in late life, accounting for at least 50 percent of all dementias, is senile dementia of the Alzheimer's type or Alzheimer's disease. Prevalence rates are difficult to obtain, but it has been estimated that 5 to 15 percent of all persons over age sixty-five and more than 25 percent of those living in nursing homes have symptoms of Alzheimer's disease. While less than 2 percent of the general population under sixty years of age are affected, rates of 20 percent or higher have been estimated for the population over eighty (Hooyman and Kiyak 1993).

The prevalence of mental disorders in old age ranges from 5 to 30 percent. Many older persons with mental disorders are treated in institutional settings rather than in community mental health services. It is suggested that approximately 5 percent of older adults are institutionalized because of psychopathological or behavioral problems (Solomon 1990). Estimates of alcoholism among older adults vary from 2 to 49 percent (Farkas 1992), and alcoholism and substance abuse are primary factors in the admission of older persons to psychiatric facilities. Schizophrenia is much less prevalent than depression or dementia in old age, and many advances in psychotropic medications have maintained current cohorts of elderly chronic schizophrenics in the community. The most common mental disorder in late life is depression, with estimates ranging from 2 to 22 percent of the population (Dunkel 1992). Manic depressive disorders are rare in old age, while unipolar depression is more common. Depression as a reaction to late-life changes is pervasive among older adults, and it is clear that depression is a risk factor for suicide. As a group, the elderly underutilize community mental health services, and treatment for mental disorders is often provided, instead, by institutionalization (Solomon 1990).

Long-Term Care Services and Costs

Planning for the future of older adults requires a continuum of care options. Until now we have emphasized institutional models of care, rather than models for community-based care. Long-term care refers to a range of services for older adults who have lost their capacity for self-care due to a chronic illness or condition and who will need care for an extended period of time. Long-term care services are provided either formally, by agencies that are paid for services, or informally, by relatives, friends, or volunteers who provide the services without compensation. Long-term care services include therapy, social services such as home care, hospice, and respite care, and rehabilitation.

Toner et al. (1993) describe current long-term care services as having three main characteristics:

—They are dominated by the Medicaid program, which stresses medical and institutional rather than community social and support services for people with chronic impairments.

—They result from fragmented federal programs, which inadequately assess the needs of persons requiring long-term care. Each program deals only with an isolated aspect of an individual need. For example, the Supplemental Security Income (SSI) program raises income above the poverty level, but neglects to address the issue of quality of life.

—Title III of the Older Americans Act and Title XX of the Social Security Act have provided opportunities for developing community services, but neither has achieved the volume of services or the specific focus on long-term care that might make such services a major element in the delivery of long-term care. (3)

Those who are the target of long-term care services include the well elderly, the temporarily ill elderly, the frail elderly living in the community, and the frail elderly living in institutions.

The data on the increased number of older adults in the population are dramatic. The numbers of institutionalized older persons are expected to continue to increase, particularly those among the oldest-old. The future status of older adults who live in the community is not yet clear, and the concept of "active versus dependent life expectancy" needs to be further explored. If, for example, older persons will be active and healthy for longer, as the research suggests, planning will require an emphasis on active lifestyle programs and services. If, however, the increased numbers of the very old will be a group of frail older persons, then the need for long-term care services both at home and in institutional settings will be very different. These differences will dramatically affect the future costs of community care and institutional care and the resources allotted to each; it is not an either-or situation.

The costs of institutional care have risen considerably since 1960. At the same time, demand for community care has also increased, but funding has not. Although gerontologists espouse the benefits of providing services to older adults in their own homes, as older people prefer, federal and state programs have not been funded to provide home care services. Long waiting lists and a shortage of home care workers are commonly found. Medicare reimbursement severely limits the number of services provided by nurses, social workers, and therapists to patients in the home. The criteria for home care services includes skilled care services and excludes the management of persons with dementia. Services that are reimbursable by Medicare are similar to those that are available in a hospital setting. Medicaid reimbursement provides somewhat better home care services allotments and even includes twenty-four-hour assistance. Yet, for community residents who are in the middle income range and not eligible for Medicaid, home care services must be paid out of pocket. The exorbitant costs of these services on a daily, weekly, or monthly basis results in their being limited to those older adults who can afford to pay for them. Thus, reimbursement remains biased toward institutional care, while policy makers continue to espouse community care as the preferred choice, to reduce the cost of unnecessary institutionalization.

THE COSTS OF INSTITUTIONAL CARE

At this time the United States spends more on health care than any other country in the world. The United States spends $600 billion annually on health, nearly 12 percent of the gross domestic product. Health services for older adults account for 36 percent of total health expenditures. Approximately 25 percent of the United States federal budget has been allocated to programs that primarily benefit older persons. The average expenditure for personal health services for persons age sixty-five and over is nearly four times that of persons under age sixty-five. At least 25 percent of older people, for example, are expected to face catastrophic illness at some point (Hooyman and Kiyak 1993). In 1984 Medicare paid 45 percent of health care expenditures for older Americans, out-of-pocket expenses were 30 percent, Medicaid 12 percent, private insurance 7 percent, and other government sources paid for 6 percent of health care expenditures.

The increased costs of institutional care can be attributed to several factors, such as the success of medical technology, the disproportionate amount of care and services needed by individuals during the last year of life, and the conflict between the curative goals of medicine and the chronic, long-term needs of older persons. The emphasis on acute, high-tech medical care has resulted in a growing demand for custodial care for the elderly, particularly for the frail elderly, and escalating long-term care costs. The rise in health care costs in the United States has been attributed to the increased needs and demands of a graying nation. Yet this issue can be debated, since the United States does not have the highest percentage of older adults in the world; only 13 percent of the population is over sixty-five years. In Sweden over 20 percent of the population is over sixty-five, and health care costs are not as high as in the United States.

The United States has developed health care and services for older adults based on a medical model that is dominated by acute crisis care. The bias in this country has been toward institutional treatment. Mental illness is still primarily treated in hospitals. Physical illnesses are also usually treated in acute care hospitals. The development of treatment facilities for the chronically ill elderly saw the growth of the nursing home industry in the 1970s. The nursing home was developed as a long-term treatment facility for the convalescent older adult then for the chronically ill, the homeless, the mentally ill, and the dying. The term *nursing home* is a misnomer: the nursing home is not a home in any sense of the word other than being a residence. It is based on a medical model and staffed with nurses to provide treatment and care. Although many attempts have been made to create a homelike atmosphere within nursing homes, still they are health care facilities based on a medical model, and they offer medical care to "patients." Regulations by the state and federal governments have been based on the medical model. Only in some states are social services and recreational activities required in nursing homes; frequently, they are referred to as "therapies," which suggests treatment as indicated in the medical model.

In the United States over seventeen thousand nursing homes are primarily funded by Medicaid (Tirrito 1993), and the reimbursement systems of Medicare and Medicaid are biased toward institutional medical services. Under the current prospective payment system, hospitals that rely primarily on Medicare are reluctant to pay for additional days for an older person and try to discharge him or her to a nursing home or private home as quickly as possible. The shape of U.S. health care is largely determined by its methods of payment, and the health care of older Americans is primarily funded by public spending—that is, by Medicare and Medicaid. Thus, public financing for health services has also meant public pressure on finding ways to reduce costs. Price inflation in the health care sector has risen faster than the general inflation rate for the last fifteen years (Hooyman and Kiyak 1993), and the costs of institutional care continue to rise substantially.

16

Medicare

In the 1980s the problem of rising health care costs became a topic of national concern. The Medicare bill was passed in 1965, and it included two parts: part A, which provided basic hospitalization insurance for those who qualify for Social Security or railroad pensions and their dependents, under certain conditions; part B, which, after paying an annual deductible and a monthly fee, covers some outpatient care, including physician services. Payments for medications, eye care, and dental care are excluded.

The Medicare program accounts for nearly 7 percent of all federal spending. When the Medicare program was initiated in 1965, it was considered a program of acute care benefits, and its annual cost was three billion dollars. In 1985 the annual cost had risen to fifty billion dollars (Hendricks and Hendricks 1986). In 1983 the revisions to the Social Security Act included the Medicare Prospective Payment Plan, and a three-year transition was planned for diagnostic-related groups, or DRGs. The DRGs are classifications used in determining payment, as indicated in the ICD-9-CM manual, which lists medical and surgical procedures. This plan was to pay hospitals a flat fee for treatment of Medicare patients as per a physician's diagnosis upon a patient's admission to the hospital. Hospitals were to be rewarded for keeping costs down and encouraging the speedier discharge of patients. In 1990 the Catastrophic Health Care Act attempted to increase Medicare benefits for long-term care by increasing the number of days of Medicare coverage for rehabilitation in a nursing home and extending the number of lifetime days of nursing home coverage provided. This act was repealed the same year (1990) by an outraged elderly constituency, whose members recognized that these changes were not in their best interests and were not needed at this time.

Medicaid

Medicaid is the means-tested federal and state program that provided access to health services to an estimated 23.6 million persons in 1987, including 12.3 million children, 3.3 million persons over sixty-five, 3 million with disabilities, and 5.8 million other adults (Kingson 1990). All states provide outpatient and inpatient hospital services, skilled nursing care, some home health services, and physician services. Variations from state to state has increased the dilemma for older adults and their families. The primary burden for the states has been nursing home care. Most patients who remain in nursing homes exhaust their savings within one year. The average annual cost of nursing home care is, nationally, thirty-five thousand dollars. Some states have costs of over sixty thousand dollars annually.

Patients who live long enough deplete their resources and must be supported by Medicaid funds. The states have been primarily responsible for the burden of nursing home costs, which have increased so dramatically that state budgets have suffered as a direct result. States such as New York, California, and Massachusetts are struggling with the high costs of nursing homes and are limiting access to nursing home beds for Medicaid patients, attempting to fill them with private pay patients, instead.

Medicaid provides funding for home health care services. States have maintained tight fiscal control over these services by limiting their eligibility for Medicaid coverage. The bias toward institutional long-term care in the United States results in large measure from the criteria used to determine eligibility under Medicaid. It is easier to qualify for Medicaid benefits as a nursing home patient than as a home care patient. The reimbursement system has created a bias toward institutionalization for older adults (Tirrito 1993). Older adults who need services and can possibly be maintained at home if services are available for ineligible Medicaid patients are placed in nursing homes, where they can receive all the services they need, such as help with dressing, bathing, food preparation, and medical care. Demonstration projects throughout the country are experimenting with Medicaid waivers for programs that provide services at home, such as the On Lok program in California.

THE COSTS OF COMMUNITY CARE

In the past ten years rising costs of nursing home care and the psychological effects of nursing home placement have prompted the government and health care professionals to search for alternative methods of providing custodial care for the chronically ill. Surprisingly, the "home" was rediscovered as a place of treatment and care. The trend toward having services in the home, or home care, has increased since 1989.

The debate continues regarding the cost-effectiveness of obtaining and providing care and treatment to older adults in nursing homes or, instead, in their own homes. The costs of institutional care have been well analyzed. The evidence has been mixed regarding the extent to which community care involves cost savings compared to institutional care (Cox 1990). Demonstration projects such as the National Long-Term Care Channeling Demonstration Program were funded by Congress in 1980. Twelve states were selected to provide a range of health and social services to long-term care clients. They provided outreach/ case finding, screening, client assessment, and case management. Some demonstration projects (e.g., the On Lok program) were designed to test alternative reimbursement programs. Efforts in several rural states permitted hospitals to provide long-term care using the "swing bed" concept of care. In addition to testing new forms of service delivery, federally funded demonstration projects have addressed problems in programs by creating waivers and merging funding streams to establish interagency planning bodies to recommend reforms in long-term care (Harrington, Newcomer, and Estes 1985). Most states, however, are cautious about funding of long-term care programs. States can control entrance to nursing homes by limiting the number of Medicaid beds. This approach has created a population of older adults and caregivers who are suffering the burdens of providing care. Hospitals are still biased toward channeling the elderly into nursing homes rather than toward community care. Discharge planning to nursing homes is more expedient than planning home care services and monitoring services to older adults in the community.

Nationally, the continuing rise in health care costs, and especially long-term care costs, has created much concern. Most states are struggling with their Medicaid budgets and are looking for solutions to the long-term care problem. Current trends in reimbursement mechanisms have not improved access or the quality of care provided to older adults in the community or in institutions. It is obvious that the long-term care dilemma cannot be solved by increasing complex reimbursement mechanisms or developing more sophisticated tools for measuring the outcomes of services. The need for collaboration at the community level is a step toward improving community care services for older adults and reducing institutional costs.

THE BIAS TOWARD INSTITUTIONALIZATION

The bias toward institutional long-term care is evident in the reimbursement mechanisms for long-term care. For example:

1. Medicare provides reimbursement for some treatments in acute care settings but not in home visits.
2. Medicare pays for physician visits, rehabilitation therapies, and skilled nursing services, such as treatments for decubitus ulcers and oxygen therapy, done in the home as an alternative to having these treatments performed in the hospital.
3. Medicare coverage in hospitals is based on the diagnostic-related groups system, and the length of stay is determined by the diagnosis and treatments ordered by the primary physician.
4. Medicare provides reimbursement for rehabilitation devices to aid in restoring the patient to a previous level of functioning.

5. Medicare provides reimbursement for hospice care for terminally ill patients for a limited period of time.

Medicaid is the primary payer for nursing home care but is limited in most states in terms of providing for home care services. Although community care has been reported to be the preferred choice of older adults, reimbursement mechanisms have not supported home care services. Basic services to maintain a client at home, such as housekeeping services, are not reimbursed by Medicaid or Medicare unless a medical diagnosis indicates that the patient is unable to manage activities of daily living due to a physical disability. Consequently, millions of people with cognitive impairments are not eligible for home care services and must be institutionalized. It is easier to place a cognitively impaired person in an institution than to provide services at home for that client; thus, institutionalization is often the answer for the older adult.

THE NEED FOR AN ALTERNATIVE PLAN

Regulations by the federal and state governments set standards for quality in nursing homes care. The need for the development of a community multidisciplinary practice approach is urgent if we are to avoid regulation of home care services. Federal and state regulations monitor physician visits in the institution (hospital or nursing home). Psychiatric services are regulated by Medicare reimbursement, which has a five hundred–dollar maximum for mental health outpatient treatments. Nursing care is regulated by allowing a limited number of patient treatments in a given time period. A patient's progress is monitored in physical therapy programs and measured in outcomes of treatment. Social worker assessments are permitted, but counseling services are not, and psychological services are seldom provided. Nursing homes are required to provide religious services in some manner. Legal services are not available to nursing home patients unless privately secured by the patient or his or her family.

It remains a much simpler task to institutionalize an older person than to arrange for services in the home. The nursing home provides housing; food; laundry and housekeeping services; nursing services; safety management; recreational activities; pharmaceutical services; physical, speech, and occupational therapy; medical services; nursing care; social services; and financial management of pensions. The medical model for reimbursement of services to the administration is easily measured and monitored. The number of meals, number of treatments, number of physician visits, and number of medications are all quantifiable. The outcomes are measured in the progress plan for each patient. The medical model was responsible for the implementation of DRGs in the hospitals and for the implementation of resource-related groups (RUGS) and minimum data sets (MDS) in the nursing homes.

There is a beginning plan for this type of linkage in home care services. Currently, Medicare and Medicaid reimbursement for home care providers has regulations for each of the professionals providing services to the client in the home. The number of nurse visits and social work visits are linked to the plan of care for the patient. Complex medical problems may justify more home care visits by the nurse, physician, social worker, home health care aide, or housekeeper. Services are based on a medical model. No such regulation yet exists, however, for the practice of independent professionals in the community.

Interprofessional collaboration has become commonplace in institutional settings but remains rare in community settings. It is imperative that professionals self-regulate and provide a continuum of long-term services in the community to better serve older adults. Methods for the development of a multidisciplinary approach will be presented in the following chapters.

REFERENCES

Chappell, N. L. (1994). Home care research: What does it tell us? *Gerontologist* 34, no. 1: 116–20.

Cox, C. (1990). Home care. In *Handbook of gerontological services,* ed. A. Monk, 2d ed., 508–27. New York: Columbia University Press.

Dunkel, R. E., and T. Norgard. (1992). Depressive disorders. In *Mental health and the elderly,* ed. F. Turner, 183–208. New York: Free Press.

Farkas, K. (1992). Alcohol and elderly people. In *Mental health and the elderly,* ed. F. Turner, 328–55. New York: Free Press.

Fries, J. F. (1980). Aging, natural death and the compression of morbidity. *New England Journal of Medicine* 303, no. 3: 130–35.

Ginsberg, L. (1992). *Social work almanac.* Washington, D.C.: NASW Press.

Gutheil, I. (1990). Long-term care institutions. In *Handbook of gerontological services,* ed. A. Monk, 2d ed., 527–46. New York: Columbia University Press.

Harrington, C., R. J. Newcomer, and C. L. Estes. (1985). *Long-term care of the elderly.* Beverly Hills, Calif.: Sage.

Hendricks, J., and D. C. Hendricks. (1986). *Aging in mass society.* Boston: Little, Brown.

Hooyman, N. R., and A. H. Kiyak. (1993). *Social gerontology,* 3d ed. Boston: Allyn and Bacon.

Kingson, E. R. (1990). Public income security programs for the elderly. In *Handbook of gerontological services,* ed. A. Monk, 2d ed., 268–97. New York: Columbia University Press.

Johnson, C. L., and L. A. Grant. (1985). *The nursing home in American society.* Baltimore: John Hopkins University Press.

Johnson, R. J., and F. D. Wolinsky. (1994). Gender, race, and health: The structure of health status among older adults. *Gerontologist* 34, no. 1: 24–35.

Katz, S., L. G. Branch, H. H. Branson, M. H. Papsidero, J. A. Beck, and J. C. Greer. (1983). Active life expectancy. *New England Journal of Medicine* 309, no. 14: 1218–24.

Monk, A. (1990). *Handbook of gerontological services,* 2d ed. New York: Columbia University Press.

National Center for Health Statistics (NCHS). (1986). Current estimates from the National Health Interview Survey: U.S. National Health Survey, ser. 10, no. 164. DHHS Publication no. 82–1569.

———. (1989). Current estimates from the National Health Interview Survey: U.S. *Vital and health statistics,* ser. 10, no. 176: 1–221.

Schneider, E. L., and J. A. Brody. (1983). Aging, natural death and the compression of morbidity: Another view. *New England Journal of Medicine* 309, no. 14: 854–56.

Solomon, K. (1990). Mental health and the elderly. In *Handbook of gerontological services,* ed. A. Monk, 2d ed., 228–68. New York: Columbia University Press.

Tirrito, T. (1993). Reimbursement mechanisms and their impact upon nursing home patients. In *Long term care,* ed. J. A. Toner, L. M. Tepper, and B. Greenfield, 42–54. Philadelphia: Charles Press.

Toner, J. A., L. M. Tepper, and B. Greenfield, eds. (1993). *Long term care.* Philadelphia: Charles Press.

Turner, F., ed. (1992). *Mental health and the elderly.* New York: Free Press.

U.S. Bureau of the Census. (1993). *Statistical abstract of the United States: 1993,* 113th ed. Washington, D.C.: U.S. Government Printing Office.

Verbrugge, L. M. (1985). Gender and health: An update on hypotheses and evidence. *Journal of Health and Social Behavior* 26:156–82.

Chapter 2

A MULTIDISCIPLINARY APPROACH
Impact on the Need for Services

A DEFINITION OF MULTIDISCIPLINARY ACTIVITY

This chapter presents a definition of multidisciplinary activity, a review of professionalization, a history of collaborative efforts, methods for collaboration, and resources for collaborative efforts. The methods used for multidisciplinary planning in nursing homes and hospitals and the current trends for case management by home health care agencies are collaborative efforts that will be discussed in this chapter. Methods of collaboration will be presented from a theoretical perspective, and new resources for the collaborative effort will be offered. In addition, the importance of community collaborative efforts by solo practitioners is discussed, including problems encountered with the multidisciplinary approach in both institutional and the community settings.

Multidisciplinary activity is not a new concept and is the foundation of the field of gerontology. Gerontology is the study of the biological, psychological, and social factors that impact the aging process. Hendricks and Hendricks (1986) describe gerontology as lying on the borders of many disciplines. Although there is no complete agreement, there is consensus that a common body of knowledge exists and that gerontology is multidisciplinary in nature. More knowledge is needed in each of the areas related to gerontology to understand the processes of aging.

The field of gerontology includes researchers and practitioners from such diverse fields as medicine, biology, nursing, dentistry, psychiatry, sociology, psychology, economics, political science, religion, social work, pharmacy, and public health. Geriatrics is a specialty in medicine, dentistry, nursing, and psychiatry which is focused on diseases of aging. The field of gerontology has experienced substantial growth since its formal development in the 1940s. The depression of the 1930s caused increased concern about older adults. After 1940

23

activity in gerontology increased dramatically. In 1945 the Gerontological Society of America was formed with a small number of researchers and practitioners who were interested in gerontology and geriatrics. Today the organization is only one of many, nationwide, and its membership is between six thousand and seven thousand.

Joint cooperative ventures among some disciplines have become customary. Medical social work had its beginnings in hospitals as physicians recognized the need to consider patients' emotions and to manage their environments if patients were to improve medically. Other disciplines such as medicine, nursing, religion, law, political science, and psychology have been reluctant to become involved in multidisciplinary activity. The era of specialization in our society has been dominant for several decades. Changes can be expected due to the complexity of problems and the scarcity of resources to manage them.

In recent years the control of health care costs has drawn national attention to community services that seem to be less expensive than institutional services. The home health care industry has proliferated. The number of home care agencies has increased from 252 in 1966 to an estimated 10,000 in 1986 (Cox 1990). Home care agencies tend to be multidisciplinary in their activity. Nursing homes began to include multidisciplinary assessments in their evaluation of patients in order to maximize the functional ability of their chronic care patients. The increase in the population of older adults and the emphasis on community services has precipitated a greater need for community professionals to collaborate in their efforts to increase the quality of their services to older adults.

Traditionally, solo community practitioners have maintained private practices. In our opinion this scenario will change. The authors present a model for solo professionals from various disciplines to practice effectively with older community adults because they believe that a multidisciplinary approach is the means to the delivery of quality services.

Collaboration is a term that has been defined in many ways. It generally refers to working together (Andrews 1990). *The Encyclopedia of Social Work* describes interdisciplinary collaboration as occurring "when different professionals, possessing unique knowledge, skills, organizational perspectives and personal attributes engage in coordinated problem solving for a common purpose" (175). In the last several decades increased specialization has led to an overlap among professionals in service delivery to various groups of clients such as children and older adults. Clients are frequently confronted with unnecessary services, overlapping services, inappropriate referrals, lack of account-

ability, and fragmentation of services (Andrews 1990). Andrews argues that the collaborative effort is affected by the characteristics of participants and the degree of shared decision making of the participants. She says, "Ideally interdisciplinary collaboration is collegial and democratic, however, professionals bring their own personalities, feelings and attitudes toward the collaborative relationship" (176). No models exist of collaboration. Some typologies exist which define collaboration along a continuum from mild to intense. Andrews describes collaboration as *multidisciplinary* when collaborators practice their independent disciplines and share information about a common case and *interdisciplinary* when collaborators mutually decide who will perform particular case functions. The authors of this book will use this definition of *multidisciplinary* to describe the approach to be used for professionals who serve older community adults; it will be used interchangeably, however, with the term *multiprofessional.*

Casto and Julia (1994) describe what they call *interprofessional care and collaborative practice,* in their book by the same title. They believe that interprofessional collaboration is a powerful tool. They define a "helping professional" as

a professionally trained person who provides professional and personal services to individuals, groups, and social systems with the intent of improving their quality of life. . . . When prevention is not possible and problems already exist, helping professionals provide assessment, encouragement, support, alternatives, and—where needed and possible—healing. (12)

Theoretical perspectives of various professions may hinder the collaborative process. When professionals recognize and develop the areas of agreement between them, however, they will realize the value of interprofessional collaboration. More and more helping professionals from various disciplines have come to recognize the person-environment fit and the systems approach, which recognizes the impact of environment and other social systems on the individual. The physician recognizes that the disease process and the healing process can be affected by the individual's environment. The minister realizes that religiosity can be impacted by the environment's social systems. Casto and Julia (1994) believe that, "even in the absence of interprofessional collaboration, a helping professional who is relationally and holistically oriented will try to be sensitive to people's multidimensionality" (18).

The terms *multiprofessional, transprofessional,* and *interprofessional* are defined as follows:

Multiprofessional suggests that more than one profession is interested in a problem;

Transprofessional indicates that professionals are engaged in work that encompasses a number of professions;

Interprofessional suggests professionals who come together to work to solve a common problem. (Casto and Julia 1994, 19)

The interprofessional approach does not blur distinctions between disciplines but, instead, works for an approach in which contributions are made to the process by the various professionals.

AN OVERVIEW OF PROFESSIONALIZATION

Professionalization is the process whereby knowledge becomes a profession. Professions are defined as having a body of knowledge, skills, and expertise (Casto and Julia 1994). Education and socialization transform nonprofessionals into professionals. Socialization is a process of developing the skills, knowledge, and behavior of a profession. Part of the process of socialization is teaching professionals to work collaboratively with their colleagues from other professions. Although some professions have not stressed collaborative work, the complexity of today's problems will demand collaboration by professionals.

Community professionals in the disciplines of medicine, psychiatry, social work, nursing, law, and religion can work together and share information. Collaboration in community practice has been nonexistent by solo professionals. Traditionally, the physician has *not* conferred with the psychiatrist, lawyer, or religious leader about the treatment plan for a client. Each practitioner develops his or her own plan, and rarely do practitioners inform one another of their treatment plan. The client may be interviewed by various professionals, with little or no communication among them and certainly no collaboration. The client's lawyer rarely contacts the person's spiritual leader, physician, or psychiatrist unless a request is made by family members or the client. It is imperative that health professionals begin to examine their roles in the community and develop methods to work effectively and collaboratively with one another. Older adults often are the recipients of fragmented service delivery that includes an overlap of services that are ineffective in providing solutions to their problems.

THE HISTORY OF COLLABORATION

Multiprofessional teams began to appear in the 1940s (Casto and Julia 1994). The complexity of chronic illnesses required the work of teams of professionals. In the 1960s multidisciplinary teams became common in the health care field, representing professionals from medicine, nursing, social work, occupational therapy, nutrition, and other health care disciplines. In the 1970s and 1980s increased federal regulation and scarce resources necessitated the multidisciplinary approach to solve various medical problems and to manage vulnerable groups of people efficiently. Interprofessional teamwork emerged in the 1970s. The interprofessional team is different from other approaches in that it "involves the interaction of various disciplines around an agreed upon goal to be achieved only through a complex integration or synthesis of various disciplinary perspectives" (Casto and Julia 1994, 36).

METHODS OF COLLABORATION

Some forms of collaboration are *conferring, cooperating,* and *consulting* (Casto and Julia 1994). Conferring refers to the informal sharing of observations. Colleagues can confer and share their opinions about a client; a physician may confer with a psychiatrist, or two psychiatrists may confer with each other about a client.

Cooperating refers to a sharing of ideas and information. This is a less formal structure of collaboration. A minister might agree to cooperate with a social worker by providing transportation via the church van for a member to attend a mental health clinic. A psychiatrist may cooperate with a lawyer and discuss with an older client the need to meet with the lawyer for estate planning.

Consulting refers to a more formal process of seeking an opinion from another professional. A physician may consult with a psychiatrist about the medication interactions of a depressed client. A lawyer may consult with a psychiatrist about the mental status of a client. In community practice all three forms of collaboration can be involved. "Teams are defined as groups of professionals that consult, confer, and cooperate formally and deliberately over a considerable period of time" (Casto and Julia 1994, 62). Teams can include various professionals, depending upon the functions and tasks of the teamwork. Some of these are:

administrator, architect, clergy, dietician, engineer, health educator, lawyer, nurse, occupational therapist, pharmacist, psychologist, physical therapist, physician, recreationist, researcher, social worker, speech therapist, teacher, vocational counselor.

The structure of teams vary according to their function. Health care teams carry the primary responsibility for delivering health care. Research teams study social or medical problems. Educational teams collaborate to teach about specific issues. Advisory boards address community problems. Professional groups are formed to study and propose solutions to national and international problems such as AIDS. All of these issues require collaborative efforts by members of various disciplines working toward a common goal.

COLLABORATIVE EFFORTS

Hospital Multidisciplinary Teams

Collaboration has been recognized as an effective practice in hospitals because team planning for patients is required there. In 1983 in the hospital system, in the early stages of diagnostic-related groups' method of reimbursement, multidisciplinary teams emerged to plan the discharge of patients in a timely manner. Teams consisting of physicians, nurses, social workers, and medical records personnel became involved in planning and assessing discharge needs in order that patients could leave the hospital as quickly as possible. Hospital teams meet regularly to discuss plans for treatment and discharge. Responsibility is shared in a collaborative process. It can be described in the continuum of collaboration as moderate collaboration in which multidisciplinary treatment teams of professionals work together to develop plans for service delivery for patients.

A more recent development in hospital care is the geriatric assessment unit. In geriatric units the importance of collaborative efforts are obvious. Geriatric assessment includes the physical, psychological, and social factors affecting a client. A multidisciplinary team conducts assessments, each from the perspective of the members' own discipline and each with its own measurement tools. Assessments are designed to evaluate functioning, to identify physical and mental problems, and to determine eligibility for programs and benefits. Unfortunately, in the context of current legislation it is functional deficiencies that serve as a criteria for need, and eligibility for services is determined on this basis. Most measurement tools used by geriatric assessment units include information from various disciplines such as medicine, psychology, nursing, social work, rehabilitation, and nutrition. Geriatric assessments require a multidisciplinary effort.

Team effort is also required in geriatric rehabilitation assessments and treatments. Rehabilitation applies methods and materials of science and technology to the process of restoring, preserving, or enhancing function or performance. Disciplines in this area include physiatry, physical therapy, occupational therapy, speech therapy, and exercise science. Geriatric rehabilitation focuses on improving the functioning of older adults with disabilities. The goal of rehabilitation is for the individual to achieve maximum fulfillment and the greatest possible independence. Team efforts are required to develop and carry through rehabilitation programs for older adults. Generally, a person with a hip fracture requires services of an orthopedic surgeon, a psychiatrist, a physical therapist, and perhaps an occupational therapist. In addition, services of a nurse, social worker, and psychotherapist may be needed to bring the person back to his or her previous level of functioning. For example, a person who has suffered a stroke will very likely require evaluation and planning by a physician, a nurse, a physical therapist, possibly a speech therapist, an occupational therapist, a social worker, and a family counselor.

As a focus of current policy efforts, geriatric rehabilitation is considered to be a measure aimed at reducing the costs of long-term care. Efforts to restore, maintain, and improve functioning in older adults requires that institutional teams (e.g., in hospitals or nursing homes) join together to plan and monitor rehabilitation programs. With a collaborative effort and modern technology much progress has been made to improve the functioning of older adults.

In treating mental illness, hospital treatment plans have developed a multidisciplinary approach. Programs are planned to meet the needs of the whole person and consider the social, educational, medical, recreational, and psychological needs of residents. Multidisciplinary work is an important aspect of mental health practice with older adults because the first plan of treatment for an older adult who seems to be mentally ill should be eliminating medical problems or sensory deficits as contributing factors. For instance, an older woman who spends most of her time arranging items in her room may be exhibiting obsessive-compulsive symptoms, or she may be compensating for visual losses. Hearing loss has been identified as a contributing factor in paranoid ideation (Davies 1992). Polypharmacy is often a contributing factor in that it can induce psychotic behaviors. In these cases appropriate review of medications by geriatric pharmacologists is necessary. Dementia can be inaccurately diagnosed. It can be the result of medications or even of nutritional deficiencies. Assessment and consultation by pharmacologists and nutritionists can prevent misdiagnosis.

Nursing Home Multidisciplinary Teams

In 1987 nursing homes adopted the model of multidisciplinary team collaboration when federal regulations under the Omnibus Reconciliation Act required the development of quality assurance programs and multidisciplinary assessments for patients in nursing homes. In this system long- and short-term

29

goals were asked to be clearly defined and measurable. Rehabilitation and discharge from the nursing home to a lesser-care facility or private home were to be considered primary goals for each patient. Objectives and "problems solutions" had to be developed for each patient by a multidisciplinary team.

Nursing home multidisciplinary teams include physicians, nurses, social workers, physical therapists, speech therapists, recreation therapists, nutritionists, and administrators. Plans are reviewed on a quarterly basis, and new measurable goals and objectives are set for each patient. This collaborative effort strives to eliminate the duplication of services and enhance the quality of care for nursing home patients. For example, the dietitian plans a specific diet for a diabetic who the physician feels is overweight or for a patient who needs a high-protein diet to heal a decubitus ulcer. A physical therapist plans the patient's therapeutic schedule with information from the social worker regarding the patient's home environment. Other benefits for clients which can be the result of collaborative team efforts for nursing home patients are included in the following cases.

CASE EXAMPLE

Jacqueline Sol is a seventy-five-year-old woman with the diagnosis of Alzheimer's disease who lives in a nursing home. She is confused and unable to bathe, dress, or feed herself. She wanders and becomes agitated when restricted to any particular area of the facility. She wanders into other patient's rooms, disturbs them and takes their belongings. The interdisciplinary team met to resolve some of Jacqueline Sol's behavior management problems. The team planned for her to become involved in recreational activities designed for patients at her level of cognitive impairment. She was to be taken for a walk outdoors each morning by a nurse aide. She was to be involved in an aerobic exercise program in the physical therapy department on alternate days. Behavioral modification techniques were to be developed specifically for her by the social worker. In addition, she was to be involved in music therapy with the recreation therapist. The problem solution methodology developed by the interdisciplinary team was very effective in managing Jacqueline Sol's behavior, and within three months the staff reported that she was less agitated than before and less hostile.

John Sol is eighty years old and is Jacqueline's husband. He is a patient in the same nursing home as she. He has multiple medical problems, including heart disease, arthritis, hypertension, diabetes, and an old hip fracture. He is unable to walk and uses a wheelchair. He can frequently be found crying, has little appetite, little interest in activities, has trouble sleeping, is often fatigued, and has expressed a wish to die. The interdisciplinary team met to formulate a treatment plan for

John Sol. The geriatric psychiatrist diagnosed the patient as suffering from a depressive disorder. Psychotropic medication was ordered and was to be evaluated regularly by the pharmacologist on the team for contraindications with the patient's other medications. The social worker was to provide counseling to resolve issues of grief regarding Jacqueline's dementia and the subsequent placement of the couple in the nursing home. The recreation therapist was to investigate John's past interests and attempt to rekindle some of his previous activities. The nurse aide was to involve him in outdoor activities each day, and the religious member of the team (in this case a priest) was to become involved in spiritual discussions with him. The multidisciplinary team's plan for John was successful, and changes were observed in his behavior within the next few weeks.

Agency Multidisciplinary Teams

Teamwork by various professionals has been successfully implemented in organizational settings. The use of group work theory has helped to improve the performance of the team. The multiprofessional team is composed of distinct professional orientations brought together to solve a variety of human problems in the human service delivery system. These varied professional perspectives offer an analysis of problems and solutions from differing orientations. The professional brings an orientation that is distinct to that professional's knowledge and training. For example, a social worker brings an ethical perspective that considers the individual as the primary concern of the team. The administrator's perspective may consider the organization its main concern. The purpose of team building is to enable work groups to function most effectively in order to benefit the client. Organizations have rediscovered the power of team effort. The formulation of ideas from each of the professions' perspectives builds a rich body of combined knowledge. Who benefits from multidisciplinary collaboration? The client benefits from the collective wisdom, professionals benefit from the support of colleagues, and society benefits from the elimination of duplicate services.

One community model of collaboration is that of case management. In home health care agencies the case manager coordinates services for clients. The first problem encountered is eligibility. The client must qualify for services. Qualification is based on Medicare/Medicaid guidelines, which dictate medical necessity for the services of the agency. Usually, home care agencies become involved in a patient's care based on a primary physician's referral. The primary physician describes which services are needed, such as nursing services, social work services, or treatment by a physical therapist and/or a caretaker at home.

The linking services of the case manager have been effective when the professionals are paid by the home care agency on a fee-for-service basis. Under the auspices of a home health care agency the services are coordinated to avoid fragmentation and duplication. This system has worked for clients who are determined to be eligible. One of the problems with this system is that the client has no autonomy: the physician and agency develop the plan of care for the patient. Another problem is that few older adults in the middle-income range are eligible.

Another type of collaborative effort by professionals from various disciplines is working with community advisory boards. Citizen participation in agency policy making has become an integral component of community organizations. What began as a generalized concept of community involvement in the planning, delivery, and evaluation of mental health services has evolved into a more specific mandate for citizen boards to ensure accountability to the community and to funding sources. The community advisory board usually insures community representation by including members of various disciplines. The multidisciplinary team or advisory board faces many of the same challenges in community work as those in institutional settings. Teamwork requires special skills and training for success.

A collaborative effort has been missing from solo professional community practice. Case management has been suggested as a collaborative effort that links older adults to community services, yet it has had limited success. The intent is to coordinate services for the client and avoid duplicating services. What is missing is the involvement of professionals who are in independent solo practice.

Establishing collaborative relationships among professionals in medicine, nursing, pharmacy, public health, and social work has been the goal of various federal and state projects. The improvement of health for rural populations is a federal goal. Various projects nationwide are under way to develop collaborative rural health programs (Macera 1993). The federal government is concerned with the lack of collaboration by health care professionals and is providing funds for encouraging collaborative efforts in preventive health care programs (Federal Register 1987). Federally supported demonstration projects under the auspices of the U.S. Health Care Financing Administration have emphasized new approaches to community care in three areas:

—the coordination and management of an appropriate mix of health and social services directed at individual client needs with the goal of reducing institutionalization and costs without sacrificing quality of care;

32

—Medicare and Medicaid coverage of long term care services in which payment for certain quasi-medical services, or changes in the location of services, may reduce the overall costs of long term care;
—innovative reimbursement methods that test whether costs are reduced without adversely affecting patient outcomes. (Harrington, Newcomer, and Estes 1985, 200)

Organized community care was implemented in a long-term care demonstration project in Wisconsin in 1974 (Harrington, Newcomer, and Estes 1985). Research has indicated the importance of interagency collaboration in many agency settings due to current legislation trends for accountability (Wimpfheimer, Bloom, and Kramer 1990). Since the 1980s agencies have been pressured by their funding sources to collaborate on programs. Scarce resources have created a climate of competition and cooperation for funds among organizations and social service agencies.

The same logic applies to community professionals. Shortages of resources and an increasing number of complex problems will require cooperation among community professionals. The importance of multidisciplinary collaboration in the community is obvious, but a model for this type of collaboration has been missing until now.

RESOURCES FOR COLLABORATIVE PRACTICE

Collaborative practice, as a means of integrated delivery of service, is a holistic approach that is gaining recognition among funding sources and in the current research. Literature in the field is increasing. Especially helpful is a new journal that began publication in the United Kingdom, the *Journal of Interprofessional Care*. This journal presents research and articles that address the holistic approach to the care of individuals in the community and in institutional settings. The Education and Human Services Consortium in Washington, D.C., has published a series of monographs on collaborative practice (Casto and Julia 1994). The National Consortium on Interprofessional Education and Practice addresses national needs from an interprofessional perspective and sponsors national conferences. The consortium stimulates the implementation of interprofessional education. Since 1978 an annual meeting is held by the Interdisciplinary Health Care Team to share information to those interested in team development in health care. An effort is being made on the national level to increase collaborative practice and develop interprofessional education. Skills needed for collaborative practice among various populations, such as children and older adults, must be researched. Baylor University in Waco, Texas, offers a program, through its College of Education, in education for collaborative practice.

Several foundations such as the Ford Foundation, the W. K. Kellogg Foundation, and the Annie E. Casey Foundation are committed to enhancing integrated service delivery. Their projects range from local initiatives to national programs for the development of new policies for integrated services. A source for identifying model programs at the local and state level is the National Center for Service Integration which serves as a clearinghouse for information and provides technical assistance to providers.

In the field of education the Ohio Commission on Interprofessional Education and Practice has made a major contribution to interprofessional learning. Other initiatives are under way at the University of Washington at Seattle and Baylor University (Casto and Julia 1994). The emphasis is on education for interprofessional practice. This book presents another effort toward educating and preparing community professionals in finding collaborative ways of integrating service delivery for older adults.

PROBLEMS ENCOUNTERED
IN THE MULTIDISCIPLINARY APPROACH

One of the problems encountered in the multidisciplinary team approach is turf conflict. Who on the team will be responsible team for preparing the treatment plan for the client? In a medical setting it is obviously a physician. In a mental health setting it is usually a psychiatrist. Authority and influence become major issues in teamwork. In hospital settings, nursing homes, rehabilitations centers, and home health care agencies authority is granted to the physician. To perform effectively groups often must overcome certain obstacles, such as:

1. confusion about roles and relationships;
2. confusion about goals;
3. lack of competence needed for the team to work effectively;
4. lack of responsibility for the task;
5. lack of a common stake in solving the problem;
6. lack of agreement about values;
7. lack of recognition of one another's expertise;
8. lack of respect for differences and opinions.

The problem of competition must be addressed. Working together on a common client system involves both cooperative and competitive elements. Cooperative work requires acknowledging the contribution of the others involved in the team effort. The prevalence of competition is all too real in collaborative efforts. Unfortunately, competitive interrelationships of practitioners can be very damaging to the client. When members fall into competitive rather than cooperative roles, the resulting situation is devastating to the purpose of teamwork. Sometimes members' ego involvement with their own professional orientations may block their ability to consider the perspectives of others. A team must remain focused on why it came together and use the expertise of the individual members to seek solutions to the given problem.

The issue of different professional orientations must be addressed. The following example indicates how professional socialization and identification foster very different views of a client's situation.

"TRAINED INCAPACITY OF SPECIALISTS"

A family may in its varied contacts receive professional care, advice, and services from a physician, a nurse, a social worker, a nutritionist, a home economist, a probation officer, a lawyer, a judge, a minister, a psychologist, a teacher, a guidance counselor, an industrial relations advisor, a banker, a group worker, and so on, each of whom may give that family irreconcilable advice and treatment, guidance in how to live, keep healthy, maintain a home and family, care for and rear children, resolve family discord, and all other aspects of living, especially human relations. The family is expected to resolve these professional conflicts, to reconcile these incongruities and often mutually contradictory advice into a coherent, consistent pattern of living, a reconciliation which a professional will not or cannot attain.

The students in medical school, nursing, social work, law, engineering, business, architecture, public administration and the graduate departments of the social sciences and humanities are being inculcated with a different conception of human nature, of human conduct, with different beliefs, assumptions, expectations about people, what and how they act and carry on their human relations. All of these students are going out to practice in our communities, with what Veblen once called the "trained incapacity of specialists" unable to communicate or collaborate in their practice or even to recognize what other specialists see and do. Indeed, we often find bitter rivalry and open conflicts arising not entirely from professional competition but from these very different beliefs and expectations, these specialized conceptions of how people act, or should act, and how they should be treated, guided and helped when in need. (Frank 1954, 89)

Multidisciplinary teams have been an integral part of the service delivery network in hospitals, outpatient clinics, nursing homes, and other health care programs. The application of this concept has been missing from community solo professional practice. The specific contributions each discipline can make must outweigh the problems inherent in the process of changing to this system. Multidisciplinary teams in community work with various populations, such as children, older adults, youth, and families, require continued research to enhance their effectiveness and training methods. Social work is familiar with the ways in which person and environment interact, and other disciplines are beginning to grasp the idea that it is essential to understand people as holistic beings. Gerontology is currently teaching other disciplines to recognize the importance of multidisciplinary activity on behalf of aging adults.

REFERENCES

Andrews, A. (1990). Interdisciplinary and interorganizational collaboration. In *Encyclopedia of social work,* 18th ed., 175–89. 1990 supp. Maryland: NASW Press.

Bargarozzi, D. A., and L. F. Kurtz. (1983). Administrators' perspectives on case management. *Arete* 8, no. 1 (Spring): 13–21.

Casto, R. M., and M. C. Julia. (1994). *Interprofessional care and collaborative practice.* Pacific Grove, Calif.: Brooks/Cole.

Cox, C. (1990). Home care. In *Handbook of gerontological services,* ed. A. Monk, 2d ed., 508–27. New York: Columbia University Press.

Davies, J. (1992). Paranoia in the elderly. In *Mental health and the elderly,* ed. F. Turner, 115–36. New York: Free Press.

Federal Register. (1987). Department of Health and Human Services. Health Resources and Services Administration. Vol. 221.

Frank, L. (1954). The interdisciplinary frontiers in human relations studies. *Journal of Human Relations* 7.

Harrington, C., R. J. Newcomer, and C. L. Estes. (1985). Long term care of the elderly. Beverly Hills, Calif.: Sage.

Hendricks, J., and D. C. Hendricks. (1986). *Aging in mass society.* Boston: Little, Brown.

Macera, C. A. (1993). *Health of the public: Community-academic partnerships—executive summary.* Report of the John A. Martin Primary Health Care Center, Winnsboro, S.C.

Wimpfheimer, R., M. Bloom, and M. Kramer. (1990). Inter-agency collaboration: Some working principles. *Administration in Social Work* 14, no. 4: 89–101.

Chapter 3

HEALTH ISSUES
Impact on the Need for Services

Good health in old age is an American dream, and in our culture the loss of one's health is a devastating phenomenon. Our society has a negative attitude toward loss of independence and the need for assistance. *Old age* and *illness* are synonymous terms in our culture. In addition to physical pain, the emotional pain of losing one's health is traumatic for older adults. The fear of not recovering to one's previous health status weighs heavily on older persons. The fear of declining health may be more troubling than the actual decline in health. The impact of health status is significantly different for older adults than for other age groups. Poor health status contributes to a host of emotional, psychological, and social problems for older Americans.

This chapter will describe the health status of older adults with an emphasis on differentiating between normal and pathological aging. The need to understand the impact of health problems upon the social and psychological functioning of older adults is reinforced. Health is presented as a central issue to well-being and psychosocial functioning. The differences between normal age changes and pathological changes must be recognized by the community professional practitioner. Diseases that are common to older adults will be discussed in order to teach practitioners to recognize their impact in planning for older adults. It is a priority that community professionals have a thorough understanding of the prevalence of diseases common to older adults and of the functional problems that may accompany them. Serving older adults effectively, whether in the community or in institutions, is not possible without knowledge of the older adult's health status.

With aging, health problems become more prevalent. Although younger people assume that older people are preoccupied with health issues, most older people consider themselves to be in good health. In a 1989 survey reported by the National Center for Health Statistics about 70 percent of older Americans in the community described their health as excellent, very good, or good, while 30 percent reported their health as fair or poor (NCHS 1986). Even institutionalized older persons tend to rate their health positively (Hooyman and Kiyak 1993). In 1987, 5.2 million persons sixty-five or older needed assistance to remain in the community. This figure is expected to reach 7.2 million by the year 2000, 10.1 million by 2020, and 14.4 million by 2050. It is projected that the proportion of persons over sixty-five years of age with one or more activity limitations will increase from the current 18 percent to 22 percent by the year 2030 (Johnson and Wolinsky 1994). It can be expected that, with this increase, health issues will become a national priority.

PATTERNS OF MORTALITY AND MORBIDITY

Social epidemiologists have used age, gender, race, and socioeconomic status to illustrate the distribution of morbidity and mortality in the United States. Recent studies have concentrated on race and gender in examining the health behaviors of older adults. Health status is the major determinant of health service delivery. Johnson and Wolinsky (1994) examined the differences in gender and race in health status and found that differences in the measurement of health exist between males and females and between blacks and whites but that the differences in the causes of perceived health exist only between males and females. Morbidity is used to predict future health service delivery needs. In older adults long-term care needs are precipitated by chronic diseases and not acute diseases.

The leading cause of death for older adults in the United States is heart disease, the second is cancer, and the third is stroke (cerebrovascular accident, or CVD). Mortality rates have decreased for deaths from heart disease and stroke. The primary reason for the decrease has been improved medical services, greater availability of coronary care units, advanced medical and surgical treatment for heart disease, improved control of blood pressure, and decreased smoking, modified eating habits, increased exercise, and healthier lifestyles among Americans (Harrington, Newcomer, and Estes 1985). Since the early 1900s there has been a substantial decrease in infectious diseases such as tuberculosis, diphtheria, and influenza as primary causes of death. Chronic diseases have replaced infectious viruses and tubercular diseases in the United States as primary causes of death. Overall, in the United States the primary cause of death are diseases of the heart.

AGE-RELATED CHANGES OR PATHOLOGICAL CHANGES

What are normal age changes, and which ones are caused by pathology? This is a subject for continued research. Dementia, for example, is a pathological condition, not a condition of normal aging condition, as myths about aging suggest. Thus, forgetfulness must be distinguished from confusion and cognitive impairment. The client who has memory lapses of events, dates, and times must be distinguished from one who is cognitively impaired and unable to remember to dress, to use the toilet or to eat. Gerontological research debates what constitute age-related changes versus pathological conditions. Many myths and a lack of knowledge still persist among professionals and older adults themselves about what is normal aging and what is pathological aging. The professional helper must be able to recognize the differences.

Health status refers not only to the individual's physical status but also to the person's functional level. Functional level refers to the management of one's daily normal activities, such as eating, dressing, toileting, walking, and bathing. Older people are more likely to suffer from chronic diseases than from acute illnesses. Yet their ability to function with these disabilities is impacted by their environment. Chronic diseases require long-term care and supportive services. The availability of supportive services, both formal and informal, is linked to the rate of institutionalization. Older adults can be maintained in their own homes with formal and informal services. The majority of older adults do live at home (95 percent). Community services can provide them with the supportive services they need to maintain their independence. Until the eradication of chronic diseases associated with old age, the health care system must be responsive to the special long-term care needs of an aging population. Treatments for diseases associated with old age are changing rapidly with advances in medical technology and the awakened interest in health promotion and disease prevention. If environmental concerns, changes in lifestyles, and new data on nutrition and stress continue to be emphasized, disability and loss of function will undoubtedly be delayed. The goal of good health in old age is a universal dream.

DEFINITION OF HEALTH

The most frequent definition of health is that of the World Health Organization (1947), which states that "health is a state of complete physical, mental and social well-being." Other definitions describe health status as the presence or absence of disease or the degree of disability in an individual's level of functioning (Hooyman and Kiyak 1993, 124). The most common term to describe one's level of functioning is *activities of daily living* (ADLs). This term refers to an individual's ability to perform personal tasks such as dressing, eating, bathing, using the toilet, walking, and getting in and out of bed. One's ability to manage his or her activities of daily living is related to that person's physical and mental health status. Mental or physical disease impairs one's ability to function, to manage these activities, and increases the risk of institutionalization.

39

CASE EXAMPLE

Angela A. was a seventy-six-year-old widow. She had been a widow for ten years. She lived alone in a senior citizen apartment complex. She fell and broke her hip five years ago. After her fall she lived with her daughter and her grandchildren for a few months. She was hospitalized several times and had many sessions of physical therapy. Her daughter was a teacher and had great difficulty caring for her mother as well as managing her home and job. Angela A. had difficulty managing her activities of daily living without help: she could not walk or use the toilet without assistance; she developed cardiac problems and had shortness of breath; and she was anxious and frightened about being alone. It was decided by her family that she would live in a nursing home, where she would have around-the-clock nursing supervision. She died three months later. The cause of death was listed as cardiac arrest. Angela A. was at great risk for institutionalization immediately after her accident. Yet, with her family support system, she was able to remain in the community for five years.

COMMON DISEASES AND CAUSES OF DEATH
AMONG OLDER ADULTS

Chronic diseases have replaced acute conditions as the greatest health risks for older adults. The most frequently reported chronic conditions in persons over age sixty-five are: arthritis (49 percent), hypertension (37 percent), hearing impairments (32 percent), and heart disease (30 percent). Other conditions among the top ten chronic conditions are orthopedic impairments, sinusitis, cataracts, diabetes, visual impairment, and tinnitus (Hooyman and Kiyak 1993).

The average older person acquires an increasing number of functional limitations resulting from age-related changes in organ systems. The incidence of mobility problems is greatest among older adults. Disease is the cause of motor disabilities, not age. Diseases such as arthritis limit mobility and may cause stiffness of the joints or difficulties with gait or posture. These are disease-related conditions and are not aspects of normal aging. Limits on mobility can be a risk factor for institutionalization for an older person who lives alone, nevertheless, as in the case of Angela A. Many impairments, however, can be managed at home.

Sensory changes frequently occur with old age. Changes in vision, hearing, taste, smell, and tactile ability are the subject of much gerontological study. Changes in vision are highly correlated with aging. Rates of impairments affecting visual functioning increase with age. There is a four times greater increase in visual impairments among those over eighty-five years than among those fifty-five to sixty-four years old. Age-related changes in the eye occur most commonly in the lens. Depth and distance perception also deteriorate with age. As a result, there is a rapid deterioration, after age seventy-five, in the ability to judge distances and depth, especially in low-light situations (Hooyman and Kiyak 1993). Many older adults are able to compensate for these losses, however, with adaptive devices and by improving environmental conditions.

Studies indicate that, in the area of auditory perception, changes in the brain are responsible for the deterioration in auditory functioning. Hearing loss also appears to be significantly related to environmental causes, such as exposure to high-volume and high-frequency noise for much of one's life (Hooyman and Kiyak 1993). Hearing loss must be appropriately assessed and diagnosed, since research indicates that older adults with hearing loss may express more paranoid ideation than they would without hearing loss. There is some clinical evidence that older persons with a diagnosis of paranoia are more likely to have severe hearing problems than are normal healthy older adults, especially those who have had hearing loss since middle age (Farkas 1990). Hearing loss must be considered in the diagnosis of paranoia. It is suggested that hearing problems can lead to social isolation and reduced intellectual functioning. It is important to note that this behavior is related to hearing problems and not to age.

A loss of taste sensitivity is no longer considered to be age associated. It was previously thought that the number of taste buds on the tongue decreased over time. Recent research, however, has challenged this notion and suggests that the number of taste buds does not decline with age (Hooyman and Kiyak 1993). Touch sensitivity is reported to deteriorate with age due to changes in the skin and partially to a loss over time in the number of nerve endings in the human body. Reduced touch sensitivity is especially prevalent in the fingers and lower extremities.

Although older adults experience age-related changes in vision, hearing, and touch sensitivity, normal aging itself does not lead to disability. It is obvious that some age-related changes can affect functioning and may require some readaptation to the environment. More research is needed to distinguish normal changes from those that are attributable to disease. Although the prevalence of disease and impairment increases with age, there is great variation in the health status of older adults.

COMMON DISEASES AND CAUSES OF DEATH AMONG OLDER ADULTS

Mortality rates indicate that the major causes of death among people over sixty-five are heart disease, cancer, and stroke (U.S. Bureau of the Census 1993). Although there has been a decline since 1968, heart disease remains the major cause of death. Since the 1960s stroke has decreased as a leading cause of death in the United States. It is estimated that eliminating cancer as a cause of death would extend the average life span by two or three years and eliminating heart disease would increase life expectancy by an average of five years and would lead to a sharp increase in the proportion of older adults in the total population (Hooyman and Kiyak 1993).

There is a gender difference in acute and chronic conditions among older adults. Men have higher rates of heart disease and cancer than women, and they have a higher incidence of fatal diseases than women. Women experience more acute and nonfatal chronic diseases than men, such as arthritis, high blood pressure, stroke, osteoporosis, and senile macular degeneration. These diseases are less likely to result in death but are more likely to reduce the quality of life for women who live to advanced old age.

CARDIOVASCULAR DISEASES

Cardiovascular diseases are among the most common sources of morbidity and mortality in old age. Hypertension is a common development that can lead to stroke, or cerebrovascular accident. The process of hardening of the arteries, or arteriosclerosis, is associated with damage to the heart, brain, and large blood vessels. The fact that most mammalian species, as they age, develop atherosclerosis (heart disease) indicates that atherosclerosis is not simply the result of intrinsic biological aging; in addition, some subpopulations in the world have been found to age to their full life spans without developing the disease (Hendricks and Hendricks 1986). Congestive heart failure is common among the older population and results from the deterioration of the heart muscle. It is often associated with edema and shortness of breath.

Stroke is a major debilitating disease for older adults and a leading cause of institutionalization; in the United States it is the fourth leading cause of death during the second half of life (Hooyman and Kiyak 1993). A stroke is the result of a cerebral hemorrhage caused by an embolism that has traveled to the brain and occluded one of the cerebral arteries or by a thrombosis that has developed in the brain's ventricular system. In both situations the brain is denied oxygen, and degeneration results. Stroke can result in the loss of speech (aphasia), paralysis on one side of the body (hemiplegia), or blindness (hemianopsia). Stroke victims require a great deal of assistance in carrying out daily activities and lengthy rehabilitation treatment by speech, physical, and occupational therapists to aid in their recovery.

Although there has been a decline in the number of deaths from stroke since 1970, it still is a significant cause of death among the elderly population. During the 1980s cerebrovascular disease was the third most common cause of death in France, Canada, and England (Hendricks and Hendricks 1986). Eighty percent of deaths from strokes occur in those over sixty-five years of age, and African-American older adults are at greater risk for strokes than white older adults. In 1987 older African Americans had twice the rate of white older adults of deaths due to stroke (Hooyman and Kiyak 1993).

Advances in technology can restore some functional ability to a disabled adult who has suffered a stroke. The process of recovery is slow and involves much assistance from formal and informal support systems; the possibility, however, of restoring a patient to functional levels has improved considerably.

Cancer

Cancer is one of the major causes of death in industrialized countries, ranking second as a cause of death in the United States, Canada, and England and first in France and Japan (Hendricks and Hendricks 1986). In the middle years, from age thirty to forty-five, women face a greater risk of developing cancer than men. Among those under thirty years of age men are at higher risk. After fifty and sixty years of age men are at greater risk than are women. Among those sixty-five and older 21 percent of deaths are due to cancer (Hooyman and Kiyak 1993). Cancer of the bowel is the most common malignancy in those over seventy years of age. Lung cancer is second in cancer-related deaths and is most prevalent among men. Lung cancer appears to be overtaking breast cancer, however, as the number one killer of American women of all ages (Hendricks and Hendricks 1986). Cancer of the colon is most common among women and rectal cancer most common among men. Older women face increasing risks of breast and cervical cancer.

Respiratory Diseases

Chronic obstructive pulmonary diseases damage (COPD) lung tissue. Their incidence increases with age, is progressive and debilitating, and often results in hospitalizations and an increased risk of institutionalization. Causes of COPD are said to be genetic and environmental (Hooyman and Kiyak 1993). Men are more likely than women to have these diseases, which have been attributed to air pollution in the community and in the workplace.

Diabetes

Insufficient insulin, which is produced and secreted by the pancreas, can lead to diabetes myelitis. It is indicated by above-normal amounts of sugar in the blood and urine, resulting from a body's inability to metabolize carbohy-

43

drates. High blood sugar levels can cause a person to enter a coma, and low blood sugar can lead to hypoglycemia, which in turn can cause one to faint. Newly diagnosed diabetes is highest among sixty- to eighty-year-olds. Adult onset diabetes is said to affect 79.7 per 1,000 older persons. Older African-American women have a higher rate of diabetes than older white women (Hooyman and Kiyak 1993). Diabetes causes excessive urination, fatigue, weakness, and slower recovery from wounds. Diabetes is a problem for older people especially because poor circulation in the extremities can lead to gangrene; in addition, when other physical illnesses are involved, it can lead to serious health problems and limitations on one's daily activities. Diabetes can be managed at home through a diet of reduced carbohydrates and calories; exercise; proper care of the feet, skin, teeth, and gums; and, for some people, monitored doses of insulin.

Accidents

A major risk for older people are accident-related injuries. Although older persons are less likely to die from accidents than younger persons, the injury is more likely to result in major functional changes in lifestyle. For example, an older person who is in a automobile accident is at greater risk for needing long-term care treatment in a nursing home than a younger person, since accidents for older person generally result in longer periods of recuperation. Rehabilitation efforts are not as vigorous as with a younger patient, and complications from the injury can develop which require nursing home care. Most of the accidents of older persons occur inside the home (Hendricks and Hendricks 1993).

ARTHRITIS AND OSTEOPOROSIS

Arthritis and osteoporosis are chronic conditions. Although it is not a leading cause of death, changes in the bones and joints which cause pain, swelling, stiffness, and a limited range of motion are major impediments to activity, and they increase the risk of institutionalization. Arthritis is an inflammation or degenerative change in a bone or joint. Since arthritis is very common among older people and symptoms are identified with the normal aging process, older people may consider its symptoms as a normal part of old age and fail to seek treatment.

Disfigurement and pain can occur in the fingers as a result of arthritis and may limit activity to a lesser extent; arthritis of the lower limbs, however, can impair mobility. Some advances in pain control and devices for enhancing mobility can be used to reduce the pain and disability of arthritic conditions. Motorized wheelchairs can improve functioning in terms of mobility. Devices for buttoning clothes and adaptive cooking and eating utensils have helped to improve functioning and to increase the independence of those with arthritis.

Osteoporosis is a softening of the bones and is particularly common among women. Hip fractures are a special problem for older women and add to their risk of institutionalization, yet recent advances in rehabilitation therapies have increased the prognosis of recovery from hip fractures. Environmental safety factors can reduce the risk of falls and fractures for older adults; indeed, preventing falls and fostering safety in the home have received much attention in the literature (Hornbrook et al. 1994). Issues of home safety, exercise, and behavioral risks were examined to develop interventions designed to prevent falls, and risk factors that contribute to falls have been studied extensively (Cummings and Nevitt 1991; Nevitt 1990; Tinetti, Williams and Mayewski 1986). A fall may be influenced by impairments that are common to older persons, such as diminished visual acuity, awkward balance and gait, or chronic diseases that may impair sensory, cognitive, neurologic, or musculoskeletal functioning. Certain drugs, especially psychotropic drugs, increase one's risk of falling. Environmental factors may play a part, including such things as poor lighting or having objects in pathways or slippery rugs. Behavioral risk factors for falls include climbing on chairs, hurrying, and running (Hornbrook et al. 1994). Falls are a major health risk for older adults.

Incontinence

A difficult noninfectious and chronic urinary problem is incontinence (inability to control urine and feces). It is estimated that incontinence occurs in 5 to 19 percent of men and 7 to 38 percent of women over age sixty-five who are living in the community. This taboo topic is of major concern for older adults and has been a major factor in the decision to institutionalize an older person. It is reported that at least half of those living in nursing homes experience at least one episode of incontinence daily. Incontinence can result from an acute illness, infection, or even medication. With age the bladder and urethra in women commonly descend, resulting in stress incontinence; with increased abdominal pressure from coughing, sneezing, or lifting, leaking can occur. Chronic functional incontinence can result from neurological changes, such as those brought on by Parkinson's disease and organic brain syndrome. Other physical causes have been reported, such as prostate problems, diabetic neuropathy, and various cancers (Hooyman and Kiyak 1993). Treatment includes drugs, dietary changes, exercises, surgical procedures, and a reduction in fluid intake. Protective products such as pads and catheters can help reduce complications and embarrassment. The following is a case example of institutionalization precipitated by incontinence.

CASE EXAMPLE

Mr. Dante, a one-hundred-year-old man, was living in his own apartment in a major city. His wife had died when he was seventy years old, and for the past thirty years he has lived in a small four-room apartment. He had two children, a son, eighty years old, living in Florida, and a daughter living nearby, age seventy-five. His daughter was widowed and in poor health with arthritis, diabetes, and a heart condition. She visited each day and shopped and cooked for him. He spent most of his day playing solitaire, watching television, and reading the newspapers. He seldom left the apartment, since walking for any length of time was tiring for him. Yet he was in good health, except for a heart condition—arteriosclerotic heart disease—which did not limit his functioning, other than to tire him out when he walked for some distance. In the past year Mr. Dante became incontinent of urine. His daughter managed to launder his clothes, but the incontinence was becoming more frequent. He occasionally had a bowel accident. He and his daughter discussed his increasing frailty and decided that placement in a nearby nursing home would be the best solution for both of them. Mr. Dante was a sensitive man and recognized that his daughter could no longer be responsible for his increasing needs.

Mr. D. was placed in Marine Nursing Home after a thorough investigation by his daughter. He had a private room. She brought a television for him, his playing cards, and had the newspaper delivered daily. Within the first week Mr. D. fell during the night while going to the bathroom. The staff became concerned for his safety during the night and asked him to call for assistance. He did not call, and so they raised his bed rails. He climbed over the rails and spoke very angrily to staff. Within this same first week he was accompanied into the shower by two nurse aides. He objected to having staff assist him with his shower and became verbally abusive and struck a nurse aide. He was referred for psychiatric evaluation, and it was determined that he was having an adjustment reaction to being placed there and was given medication to calm him down. During the second week he became lethargic and had a poor appetite. He did not communicate and was placed in a wheelchair and toileted and fed. In the third week he was not eating and was sent to the hospital since, dehydrated and needing intravenous feeding. He died on the trip to the hospital. Mr. Dante had lived successfully in the community for one hundred years but died in a nursing home within three weeks.

FUNCTIONAL LIMITATIONS

The older person's ability to function independently is based on his or her physical and mental health status. The loss of independence is of primary concern to older adults. The need for assistance with bathing, dressing, eating, walking, and toileting is not a consequence of old age but, rather, a result of illness and disability. Frailty is a threat to older adults.

Chronic medical conditions such as arthritis can lead to severe functional limitations. If chronic medical conditions can be prevented or treated effectively, it may be possible to reduce the incidence of severe functional limitation. Persons with cerebrovascular disease, arthritis, and coronary heart disease are at greater risk of severe functional limitation. Functional limitation affects the quality of one's life, increases the likelihood of hospitalization, and decreases his or her chances for survival. Functional limitation is also a major reason that supportive services such as home care and nursing home care are needed.

Technology has provided our society with many assisting devices that can compensate for disabilities among humans and help with their functional limitations. Physical therapists teach clients to use walkers, wheelchairs, commodes, hoyer lifts, three-pronged canes, and prosthetics. Occupational therapists teach clients to use devices to button clothing, open equipment, cook, and manipulate objects. Many assistive devices are available for the visually impaired and the hearing impaired. Supportive community services can enhance the frail elderly person's functioning in the home and reduce his or her risk of institutionalization.

TECHNOLOGY AND MEDICAL ADVANCES

In the last few decades medical knowledge has advanced rapidly. Technological advances have increased life expectancy and reduced morbidity and mortality. Refinements in prosthetic devices for hip fractures have improved the quality of life for older adults, and the availability of prostheses for limbs has strengthened the functional abilities of many older adults. Visual aids and hearing aids assist those with impaired eyesight in adapting the environment to their own needs. Stroke victims are able to recover some functional ability with the help of speech therapy, occupational therapy, and physical therapy. Certainly, pacemakers, angioplasty, and heart surgery extend the lives of patients with cardiovascular diseases. Medications control diabetes, eliminate pneumonia as a killer disease, and control psychiatric disturbances. Technology has also extended life with such things as feeding tubes and respiratory systems.

Yet advances in technology have brought with them certain ethical issues that need to be examined. In our society we have valued finding cures and restoring functioning for those who are ill or disabled. Medical professionals learn to spare no effort in keeping a patient alive. More and more health professionals are asking the question of whether dying should be prolonged indefinitely when there is no possibility that a patient will recover.

At this time three powerful professions—medicine, law, and ethics—are faced with the task of clarifying the definition of death and the rights and obligations of all who are involved in the decision-making process in cases of a dying patient. In the medical model aggressive treatment is the chosen method. There is increasing public support, however, for individual decision making regarding life-sustaining treatments, as evidenced by the growth in the number of persons who have living wills. Most states have initiated health care proxy legislation, which permits an individual to advise a hospital's or nursing home's administration about his or her choice of treatment in sustaining and prolonging life. Who should make decisions to maintain or end life? These decisions, and their payments—financial, physical, and emotional—are being made by older adults and their families more and more frequently. The community professional practitioner can help with these difficult decisions.

Who should receive costly surgery such as organ transplants and kidney dialysis? Oregon has passed legislation to stop spending Medicaid funds on costly transplants for a select number of patients (Hooyman and Kiyak 1993). In England there is agreement among physicians, the public, and government that equal access to health care services is more important than widespread access to high-technology services such as kidney dialysis or coronary artery bypass surgery.

Another question our society must answer has to do with what kinds of economic burdens it is willing to bear to ensure adequate health care for all older adults.

IMPLICATIONS OF HEALTH ISSUES FOR COMMUNITY PROFESSIONALS

It is essential that social workers, lawyers, religious leaders, and other non-medical professionals who work with older adults recognize the impact of health status on these people's sense of well-being and their psychosocial functioning.

The literature reviews some strategies that people use to manage illness on their own (Stoller and Gibson 1994). Health surveys suggest that many symptoms are treated outside the formal medical care system. Many of those who seek medical attention have already treated themselves before seeking medical care. Common strategies include use of over-the-counter medications; use of previously prescribed medications; use of someone else's medications; use of appliances such as heating pads or enemas; use of salves, gargles, or herbs; and a change of behaviors, such as getting additional bed rest. Women most frequently are providers of lay health care (Stoller and Gibson 1994). Men and women talk over their health problems with each other and with friends, and they share health-related information and practices. The use of lay, or folk, remedies are more common among ethnic minorities but not limited to them. A range of treatments has been identified in a New York study which included cranberry drinks for urinary problems; heating pads and liniments for muscle pain; various gargles for sore throats; and leisure activities and prayer for depression (Stoller and Gibson 1994). The needs of a healthy older adult are very different from that of a frail older adult. Understanding the physical health problems of an older person is necessary in making an accurate assessment of that person's situation. Misinterpretation of symptoms can lead to a duplication of services as well as inappropriate placements. An older adult who is experiencing hearing loss might, for example, exhibit symptoms of paranoia. The inability to distinguish words and sounds prompts misinterpretation and confusion for someone with an undetected hearing loss.

Dietary and nutritional problems can also contribute to cognitive impairment and indicate dementia. Referral to a psychiatrist is usually inappropriate until an accurate assessment is completed. Dementia has been related to nutritional deficiencies, medications, and physical illness. Reversal of this condition is possible when it is detected. Institutionalization is inappropriate.

New data suggests that there is a linkage between physical illness and depression (Caine, Lyness, and King 1993). The 1993 study by Cain and his colleagues identifies medical conditions as a possible cause of depressive symptomatology. Society's inability to compensate for role losses and ageist attitudes contributes to loneliness and depression. Some societal factors may be responsible for depression, but new studies are examining data from other contributing causes such as physical illnesses. Additional research is needed in this area before definitive conclusions can be made. Nevertheless, a community professional who is aware of these linkages would avoid unnecessary psychiatric hospitalization for the older person by investigating all of the possible contributing factors affecting a depressed person.

COLLABORATION AMONG COMMUNITY PROFESSIONALS

Recognizing that lawyers, for instance, are not trained to be geriatricians and religious leaders are not trained to be social workers, the authors have developed a screening instrument that can be used by various community professionals to accurately assess a client's physical and mental health status, not for the purpose of diagnosing and treating but, rather, for referral to appropriate services. For example, a person who is depressed may seek solace from a religious counselor before seeking psychotherapy from a mental health agency; likewise, an older adult is more likely to seek help from a religious counselor than from a mental health clinic. But does the religious counselor recognize the differences between one's need for solace and psychiatric disturbances? Can this professional accurately assess the needs of his or her older parishioner or client?

The lawyer who interviews a client for financial planning should have some understanding of the client's cognitive status. For example, if a client tells a lawyer that someone is trying to steal his or her money, the lawyer must determine whether the client is presenting an accurate situation or if there are contributing factors to this person's having made such a statement. What is the impact of physical or mental problems on the client's behavior? As discussed previously, hearing loss can be related to paranoid ideation. Thus, an attorney will want to determine whether the client has in fact been the victim of financial abuse or if hearing problems have perhaps contributed to a misunderstanding between the client and his or her significant others. In another situation, if a client appears to be suffering from dementia by providing inappropriate answers to questions or having difficulty remembering facts, is the attorney capable of determining whether a conservator should be appointed to handle the client's finances? Should the client be referred to a physician to assess his or her physical condition? Does the attorney know that several factors can contribute to cognitive impairment? It is imperative that community professionals have knowledge about the health issues affecting older adults in order to help them deal effectively with problematic situations.

Physicians maintain primary responsibility for patients in hospitals, nursing homes, and at home. If an older person presents symptomatology of depression or anxiety disorders, the physician may prescribe medication to alleviate the symptoms. Rarely does the physician recommend psychotherapy for older adults, which sometimes results in a patient using psychotropic medication for an extended period and then experiencing complications from prescribed medications. Some medications are contradictory in the older adult, and some may promote coronary dysfunction.

Linkages between professionals in planning the best treatment for an older person, though vital, is currently missing in community care.

REFERENCES

Caine, E. D., J. M. Lyness, and D. A. King. (1993). Reconsidering depression in the elderly. *American Journal of Geriatric Psychiatry* 1, no. 1 (Winter): 4–20.

Cummings, S. R., and M. C. Nevitt. (1991). Risk factors for fall-related injuries and long lives: Findings from a prospective study. In *Reducing frailty and falls in older persons,* ed. E. Weindruch, C. Hadley, and M. G. Ory, 90–95. Springfield, Ill.: Charles C. Thomas.

Gutheil, I. (1990). Long term care institutions. In *Handbook of gerontological services,* ed. A. Monk, 2d ed., 527–46. New York: Columbia University Press.

Harrington, C., R. J. Newcomer, C. L. Estes, et al. (1985). *Long term care of the elderly: Public policy issues.* Boston: Sage.

Hendricks, J., and D. C. Hendricks. (1986). *Aging in mass society,* 3d ed. Toronto: Little, Brown.

Hooyman, N., and A. H. Kiyak. (1993). *Social gerontology,* 3d ed. Boston: Allyn and Bacon.

Hornbrook, M. C., V. J. Stevens, D. J. Wingfield, J. F. Hollis, M. R. Greenlick, and M. G. Ory. (1994). Preventing falls among community-dwelling older persons: Results from a randomized trial. *Gerontologist* 34, no. 1: 16–23.

Johnson, R. J., and F. D. Wolinsky. (1994). Gender, race and health: The structure of health status among older adults. *Gerontologist* 34, no. 1: 24–35.

National Center for Health Statistics (NCHS). (1986). Current estimates from the National Health Interview Survey: U.S. *National health survey,* ser. 10, no. 164, DHHS Publication no. 82–1569, 1987.

———. (1989). Current estimates from the National Health Interview Survey: U.S. (1989). *Vital and health statistics,* ser. 10, no. 176, 1990, 1–221.

Nevitt, M. C. (1990). Falls in older persons: Risk factors and prevention. In *The second fifty years: Promoting health and preventing disability,* ed. Institute of Medicine, 5. Washington, D.C.: National Academy Press.

Stoller, E., and R. C. Gibson. (1994). *Worlds of difference.* Thousand Oaks, Calif.: Pine Forge Press.

Tinetti, M. E., F. T. Williams, and R. Mayewski. (1986). A fall risk index for elderly patients based on number of chronic disabilities. *American Journal of Medicine* 80:429–34.

U.S. Bureau of the Census. (1991). *Statistical abstract of the United States,* 111th ed. Washington, D.C.: U.S. Government Printing Office.

Chapter 4

MENTAL HEALTH ISSUES
Impact on the Need for Services

PREVALENCE OF MENTAL HEALTH PROBLEMS

The prevalence of depressive and cognitive mental disorders among older adults is well documented in the literature. The incidence of Alzheimer's disease increases with advancing age, with 25 percent of the over-eighty-five age group being affected. Similarly, the incidence of depression increases with advancing age. The increase in depression generally is related to the losses associated with aging—for example, retirement or loss of a spouse or friends. Depression afflicts a higher percentage of older women than older men. Somatoform disorders (e.g., hypochondriasis) are also likely to manifest themselves more frequently among the elderly, partly as a function of older people's increased potential for self-absorption and reduced sphere of outside activities. Substance abuse is not a disease of old age; involuntary polypharmacy is greatly evidenced among the elderly, however, with serious implications for mental functioning. Psychoses such as schizophrenia and manic depression are not more prevalent among the aged, although thought disorders are associated with organic cognitive disorders, such as Alzheimer's disease. In addition, there is a higher incidence of language disturbance (e.g., aphasia, or the loss of the ability to speak) within the elderly population. Impairment in language comprehension and ability to speak are also increased in this age group as a result of stroke, or cerebrovascular accident.

This chapter identifies the primary types of mental health problems experienced by the elderly, including depression, the major dementias, delirium, language disturbances, somatoform disorders, and substance abuse. These disorders are associated with aging and are either functional (nonbiologic) or organic in origin. The chapter will highlight those problems that are most likely to be present in the community practice situation. Special attention is given to distinguishing among the many signs and symptoms of these disorders to aid in differential diagnosis. Specific psychotherapeutic and drug treatments will also be delineated. The chapter provides a methodological framework for counseling the elderly. It will conclude with a discussion of the implications of those mental health problems requiring comprehensive assessment to determine the older person's service needs.

Depression

There are two major types of depression: endogenous, internal depressions and reactive depressions. Some individuals are generally depressed; the root of their depression might be traced to early childhood deprivations or other early experiences. Depression may also be a result of biological predeterminants, for example, compromised efficiency of norepinephrine and serotonin, which are chemicals that affect the brain's emotional regulatory system. Other individuals understandably become depressed in reaction to a loss, such as the death of spouse, retirement, or a prolonged illness. The latter group will generally recover following an expected period of emotional support.

Reactive depression is the type primarily associated with aging, although it is critical that biological and characterological influences be separated. As everyone ages, the opportunities for depression increase as a result of inevitable losses. Furthermore, depression can reflect a wide variety of medical disorders especially among the elderly (Caine, Lyness, King 1993, 4.) The incidence of depression is greater for women than men throughout the life cycle. The higher risk for women generally has been associated with their lower social status. *Involutional melancholia,* an archaic term, is still occasionally applied to depression in women who have reached or passed the age of menopause. There is no evidence, however, to support the conclusion that depression at the age of menopause is distinct from those depressions occurring at other stages of life. A major, or severe, depression at any age can be linked to either endogenous or internal factors.

The signs of depression are many, and they cover a great range. Among them, commonly, are sleeplessness, loss of appetite, generalized fatigue, apathy, decreased concentration, and selective memory loss. In addition, individuals often complain of helplessness, hopelessness, suicidal ideation, hypochondriasis, overcompliance, feelings of general dislocation, and poor or no self-esteem.

Common treatment strategies include traditional psychotherapy, often used in combination with psychotropic drugs. The most commonly used medications are the tricyclics (e.g., Elavil, Tofranil, Norpramin, and Pamelor) and Prozac and Zoloft. The MAO inhibitors (e.g., Nardil and Parnate), another group of antidepressants, are less commonly used because of possible negative interactions with other medications and dietary substances.

Somatoform Disorders

There are different types of somatoform disorders, but their common feature is an exhibition of physical symptoms with or without organic damage. A functional somatoform disorder is a physical disturbance of tissue or organ, but it is a disturbance with no damage. The patient who complains of loss of movement in an arm or leg with no physical basis is likely suffering from a conversion reaction. A psychosomatic disorder is one in which the individual exhibits physical symptoms with underlying organ damage, as in the case of ulcers or colitis. The hypochondriacal individual worries, often without any basis, about impending physical loss or injury.

An older person is likely to channel anxieties into somatoform disturbance as a result of fears of dependency and increasing frailty. In addition, if an older person can attribute problems in functioning to a physical cause, he or she is absolved of the responsibility of confronting the source of distress. The individual is also relieved of any personal sense of inadequacy, since, after all, the problem is one of a physical nature and cannot be helped.

Somatic disorders can serve a variety of defensive functions, including retribution for guilt, inhibition of angry impulses, and imposition of control over others; they are common among older people as a result of the growing likelihood that they will become more dependent on others and more limited in their social activities. These and other disturbances, such as anxiety and depression, will only become chronic in those individuals with biological and/or characterological predispositions toward them. It is necessary to evaluate the given condition, taking into account the older person's personal and work history and personality structure. Certain medications can be useful in treating the underlying anxiety or depression, including the benzodiazepines (e.g., Valium, Xanax, Ativan) and Prozac, which is effective in managing not only endogenous depression but also obsessive impulses. Many individuals can be helped through task-centered psychotherapy, in which they are helped to reengage with society in meaningful ways. It is important to recognize the extent to which loss of role and function is involved with aging in our society in identifying sources of psychopathology among older people.

Alzheimer's Disease and Related Dementias

Alzheimer's Disease is a type of dementia (cognitive, or brain, dysfunction) which involves reduced intellectual functioning, with impairment in judgment; abstraction; memory; orientation to time, place, and other people; and language disturbance. Although many conditions are known to produce symptoms characteristic of dementia in the elderly, two of them account for approximately 85 percent of all dementia occurring in persons age sixty-five and over: these are Alzheimer's disease (AD), which occurs in over 50 percent of those individuals presenting symptoms of dementia in this age group; and Multi-Infarct Dementia (MID), which occurs in 10 to 15 percent of the individuals displaying these symptoms. MID is considered to be a result of small strokes in the brain; the cause of Alzheimer's disease is not as well understood. It is thought that the condition is related to two factors: one, an abnormal buildup of a protein called amyloid, which appears to be connected with the second factor, a dysfunction in the manufacture of the enzyme that catalyzes the production and release of the neurotransmitter acetylcholine. There also seems to be some evidence of a genetic link to early-onset familial Alzheimer's disease (Travis 1993, 828). Recent genetics research has shown that a variant of a gene that allows the manufacture of one form of cholesterol-carrying protein is a major risk factor for late-onset Alzheimer's. Aluminum, once thought to be a cause of the disease, has been ruled out as a linkage to plaques, material resulting from dense protein synthesis outside the brain cell, but not necessarily to neurofibrillary tangles. Tangles are abnormal protein fibers within the brain cell which are found in Alzheimer's patients (Hendricks and Hendricks 1986, 239).

Alzheimer's disease and MID differ in that the former is characterized by a slow onset, whereas MID occurs more abruptly. In addition, the early symptoms of AD include errors in judgment, a decline in personal care, and problems with memory. The early symptoms of MID are generally evidenced by dizziness, headaches, decreased mental and physical vigor, and sudden attacks of confusion. The progress of the two conditions also vary: MID is characterized by uneven, erratic development, while with AD one will see a steady and progressive decline.

Certain dementias are reversible and, therefore, are not really dementias at all; more correctly, they are states of delirium. The onset of a delirium is acute and is exhibited by various mental function deficits. These include fluctuating memory disturbances and impairment in one's perception, coherence, and orientation. Acute confusion, or delirium, can be brought on by a host of different factors, such as drugs, emotional trauma, metabolic disease, visual or hearing disorders, nutritional deficiency, head trauma, tumor, infection, or alcohol abuse.

Furthermore, it is important to distinguish between age-associated memory impairment (AAMI) and dementia. It is estimated that 25 to 50 percent of all people over age sixty-five may experience some memory loss, particularly diminished ability to recall names, specific words, or the location of objects.

Dementia, however, involves much more severe memory loss than is experienced by those individuals with age-associated memory impairment.

Dementia, delirium, and depression are characterized by many of the same features, which, therefore, makes careful screening imperative. One clue to distinguishing a state of depression from a cognitive dysfunction is that the depression is primary; secondary deficits are reflected in loss of will, not ability. Additionally, in depression, memory loss is selective, whereas the individual experiencing dementia will exhibit global deficits in judgment, abstract thinking, memory, comprehension, orientation, and language. The depressed person is more likely to appear hopeless and noncompliant than the individual with dementia. An individual who suffers from dementia is likely to try to cover up deficits in mental capacity. Depression, in the early stages of dementia, follows from the recognition of one's increasing cognitive incapacity.

Drugs are used to manage the behavioral symptoms of dementia (e.g., depression, agitation, and sleep disorders), yet certain behaviors, such as repetitive screaming, moaning, and pacing, are not very responsive to drug treatment. Physical restraint is no longer routinely used in skilled nursing facilities because it has not been effective in reducing the incidence of falls and injuries among those suffering from dementia. There is no effective drug treatment for Alzheimer's disease; however, agents that significantly retard the degeneration of nerve cells are expected to dominate the market after the year 2000 (Lamy 1993, 95). Therapies that focus on reality orientation and reminiscence either individually or in groups are two behavioral psychotherapeutic approaches that are effective in optimizing a dementia patient's cognitive functioning and maintaining his or her socialization. Since the management of dementia is very much a family affair, family therapy approaches are often recommended in providing family caregivers with assistance in helping patients through the degenerative stages of the disease. Early-stage dementia patients need counseling and support to cope with their recognition of their cognitive losses and with their resulting anger and fear.

Language Disorders

Language disorders are most likely to be encountered among the institutionalized elderly; the vast majority of these individuals are hearing impaired and have moderate-to-severe communication impairment secondary to dementia. Changes in nursing home reimbursement policies, however, have resulted in a shift in the locus of care from the institution to the home for many individuals requiring moderate levels of care. These changes, coupled with the growth in the over-eighty population, suggest that more individuals with hearing and language deficits will be seeking mental health services from community practitioners.

There are different causes of language impairment, including hearing loss, stroke, degenerative neuromuscular disease (such as Parkinson's disease), dementia, depression, laryngectomy, and tracheostomy. *Aphasia* is the term used to describe an inability to deal with all aspects of symbolic language and is usually the result of injury or damage to the left hemisphere of the brain. It can be receptive, expressive, or both. Receptive aphasia is when one has difficulty understanding spoken and written language; expressive aphasia is when one has difficulty conveying thoughts through speech and writing.

The mental health practitioner must be very observant in identifying those functions that are still healthy in an aphasic individual and then "pitching to his or her strengths." In other words, if a patient cannot understand what one is saying, then one should use another means of communication. Holding a hand can communicate more empathy and understanding than words. If an individual is trying to say something that his or her health care worker does not understand, the professional should look for other cues that could convey the patient's intent—for example, a facial expression or gesture or something they have drawn in a picture. The practitioner must eliminate frustrating situations whenever possible, never pushing or being unreasonably demanding of the aphasic individual. The tone of voice one uses and his or her approach are particularly critical in establishing a nonthreatening environment for an exchange with the patient. If the aphasic individual is accompanied by a family member, the practitioner should attempt to communicate directly with the cognitively impaired individual, rather than talking about the patient as if he or she is not present.

An individual's inability to hear or communicate can only increase his or her sense of isolation and may result in suspiciousness and even paranoia. It is incumbent upon the mental health practitioner to reduce the opportunities for isolation and frustration. This can be done by being aware of the many available forms of expression and communication.

POLYPHARMACY

Polypharmacy is a term that describes the concurrent intake of more than one drug for single or multiple health problems. Polypharmacy arises from either involuntary or voluntary misuse of drugs. Most polypharmacy among the elderly is involuntary. The elderly population is at increased risk for this type of drug misuse, since many older people have at least one chronic condition (e.g., hypertension or diabetes), for which drugs might be prescribed. In addition, the types of diseases (e.g., renal disorders) most frequently experienced by older people, such as renal disorders and hyperthyroidism, can contribute to altered drug responses and increased sensitivity to the interaction of certain classes of drugs. Furthermore, aging itself is associated with changes in the rates of excretion of certain drugs, which leads to increased blood levels, or heightened amounts in the blood. There are many different types of polypharmacy, which simply result from a variety of drug interactions. The present discussion focuses on those factors that may contribute to the incidence of harmful drug interactions in the treatment of certain mental conditions.

Many drugs influence functional systems. Two or more concomitantly administered drugs may affect the same systems; therefore, it is important to consider side effects. Polypharmacy has three potent effects:

1. Drugs that are "antagonists" inhibit the effects to be achieved.
2. Drugs that are "additives" increase the pharmacological effect.
3. Synergistic drugs can cause the most dangerous situations. They do not work in a 1 + 1 = 2 mode; instead, the effect can be 1 + 1 = 4 or 5 or 6, thus accelerating pharmacological reaction, which can lead to toxicity.

So with regard to the "synergistic" category of drugs. Tricyclic antidepressants and cardiotonic medications such as digoxin (from the digitalis group) can cause serious irregular heart rhythms, or arrhythmias. The patient then must be hospitalized. Twenty percent of all hospital admissions are a result of therapeutic misadventures.

It is not uncommon for an older person to take diuretics. These individuals need to be admitted to a care facility or a hospital in order to be weaned to proper drug levels, and only then are they able to resume correct therapy with drugs administered at proper dosages.

One problem that must always be taken into account is that physicians, in trying to help their patients, may inadvertently mix drugs. Too often they do not have sufficient knowledge of the other medicines that a patient is taking. Not all elderly people are reliable reporters; they are not always able to remember what drugs they are currently taking or which ones they did not take today, yesterday, or the day before. Many have family members who do not know what medications the patient is supposed to take. and many have no family at all.

If a patient does not know what medications to take, what the doctor prescribed, and for what ailment, the complications could be endless, unless the patient has a good doctor as well as a good advocate, who will make sure there is adequate follow-up.

HOW DO DRUGS WORK? WHERE THE NEW
PSYCHOPHARMACOLOGY IS HEADED

To understand, briefly, about the current drugs being used to alter mood and behavior, one must understand how the brain responds to drugs chemically. The greatest breakthrough in this area revolves around something called a neurotransmitter. A neurotransmitter is a chemical that is synthesized by a cell. The central nervous system has the ability to alter the function of the native cell and, when it is transmitted it, can change the function of cells distant from the cell of origin. A neurotransmitter is a biologically active chemical having all the characteristics of a hormone.

Neurotransmitters

There are three major neurotransmitter systems in the brain associated with normal cognitive function: dopamine, serotonergic, and adrenergic. Although "senile dementia" of the Alzheimer's type is associated with an altered cholinergic system (releasing or stimulated by acetylcholine), it is limited to this syndrome. In a similar manner L-dopa is the neurotransmitter that is altered in Parkinson's disease. Both the major neuropsychiatric clinical states respond to drugs modulating serotonin, dopamine, and epinephrine (adrenaline). To complicate matters, certain hormones and nutrients can affect these neurotransmitters. It is the ratio of neurotransmitters to one another which is critical to normal functioning.

Receptors and the Brain

Receptors either receive a signal to make neurotransmitters or, if these signals are blocked by drugs, the cell stops making neurotransmitters. Drugs can enhance or stimulate the receptors' ability to make neurotransmitters, or they can increase the cells' ability to absorb those neurotransmitters already made. This aspect of neurotransmitters only becomes more complex with other variables added.

Drugs and the Central Nervous System

Drugs that act on the central nervous system (CNS) must gain entry into the brain cell that is functioning abnormally. This is accomplished when the drug molecule is bound at the receptor site on the cell membrane. Once this is done, the complex allows for the drug to be pulled into cells where the work will take place. An example is the drug Clozapine, used for chronic schizophrenia, which acts on dopamine but also acts on the other neurotransmitters as

59

well. Understanding this is in itself a breakthrough in treating this syndrome. Obviously, the way drugs interact with the central nervous system is highly complex.

The importance of taking a thorough drug history and carefully monitoring the patient's drug therapy is now obvious. Every good clinician will have to be thorough in this regard.

Alcohol Abuse

Alcoholism is not a disease that afflicts the elderly in any great proportion. Nevertheless, it is worth reviewing some of the problems associated with alcohol abuse, since they can be confused with the symptoms of other more common organic syndromes. Furthermore, the association between depression and alcoholism portends unfavorably for women. Increased life expectancy places women at even greater risk of suffering emotional and physical losses than in prior generations. The breakdown in traditional taboos, which restricted women's involvement in the alcohol and illegal drug alcohol cultures, has likely fostered an increase in alcohol misuse among older women.

At present, between 8 and 15 percent of the elderly have serious alcohol problems. The population of elderly alcoholics is primarily male, with older men constituting 8 percent of the group and older women only 1 percent. The incidence of problem drinking is twice as high among men age twenty-one to thirty-nine. There are two types of alcoholics: those who have had a lifelong problem and those who have started drinking with the onset of old age. The majority of alcoholics have suffered from the illness their entire lives. People who become alcoholics late in life are usually responding to depression or boredom associated with changes in their lives such as widowhood or physical decline. Significant effects of lifelong alcoholism are seen in liver damage and the impact on the central nervous system. Detoxed alcoholics show significant evidence of organic brain syndrome, including deficits in sensory motor performance, perceptual capability, conceptual shifting, visual-spatial abstracting abilities, and memory function. One of the most devastating aftermaths of chronic alcohol abuse is Korsakov's psychosis (also known as Korsakov syndrome). In their early phase, or what is known as Wernicke's encephalopathy, neurological deficits first become apparent. In full-blown Korsakov's psychosis the patient exhibits severe amnesia, a tendency to confabulate and invent stories and information to cover memory deficits, and remarkable personality changes characterized by passivity, indifference, and lack of affect. A careful drug and alcohol history is obviously essential in differentiating Korsakov's psychosis from

Alzheimer's disease. The best treatment for Korsakov's psychosis or any potential complication of alcohol misuse is prevention when and wherever possible.

PSYCHOTHERAPEUTIC TREATMENT MODALITIES

The literature provides ample description of the various psychotherapeutic treatment modalities, such as the psychoanalytic, cognitive-behavioral, family therapy, or systems theory. The distinctions among these approaches will depend on one's perceptions of the client or client system. The psychotherapeutic modality is a composite of different approaches. This eclectic conception assumes that different precepts from each of these approaches are applicable when counseling the elderly at different phases of treatment; it also assumes that consideration will be given to the individual's functional age, biopsychosocial situation, and organic deficits.

A MODEL FOR COUNSELING OLDER ADULTS

The Entry Phase

The entry phase of treatment is marked by two significant activities. The first involves making a biological, psychological, and social assessment of the client (patient), and the second involves establishing a contract with the client which defines the scope of the work to be done together.

The Functional Age Assessment

The therapist or counselor takes a complete medical history and conducts an assessment of the patient's functional capabilities and limitations in managing the activities of daily living. In addition, the range of the patient's informal and formal support systems is assessed. Based on knowledge of the patient's network of family and/or friends, the therapist will be able to review opportunities for meaningful involvement by them. The patient's recent past losses must also be evaluated. Then a meaningful comparison can be drawn between the individual's experience and that of a typical age cohort member to see how the individual is faring relative to his or her peers. If the individual is functioning on the social level of the average eighty-year-old but is only sixty, this disparity provides a clue to other potential dysfunctions, including possible organic disturbances. In addition, knowledge of the informal and formal systems in which the individual is engaged provides an understanding of the importance of the family as well as of gaps in the individual's formal support system. The therapist's work with an older person is comprehensive and must include a focus on mediating the exchange between the patient and his or her informal and formal support systems. In other words, the therapist must be prepared to get involved in the life of the older person and help to coordinate his or her activities.

The individual's psychological profile should include an assessment of current obstacles and conflicts (intrapsychic and environmental). This profile includes a description of the nature of any psychological defenses present in the patient (lower-level ones such as denial or projection versus higher-level ones such as rationalization and sublimation). The nature of the anxiety—free-floating, rigidly bound, or unconscious—and the type of depression (lifelong or reactive) should also be included in the profile. Also critical in assessing the patient is the nature of his or her object relations (are they self-gratifying? mutually gratifying?). In other words, the patient's character structure should be assessed so that a particular problem is placed in a meaningful context. If a patient's husband died two years ago and she is still in a state of acute bereavement, a personality assessment will reveal whether or not she has a characterological tendency for depression. This kind of information can be useful in separating biological and social factors from psychological influences. Furthermore, the therapist can determine if the individual is struggling with developmentally appropriate conflicts, such as issues of retirement, physical aging, or perhaps spiritual concerns. Sometimes there will be conflicts representing lifelong battles with dependency on others.

The Contract

The contract represents an agreement or understanding between patient and therapist of the treatment plan to be implemented based on the patient's needs and goals. The contract also serves to provide a clear statement of expected tasks of both the therapist and the patient; it focuses the work ahead. The contract is specific; it can be limited to a certain period of time or open-ended, depending on the nature of the tasks to be undertaken. Helping a person to come to a decision regarding the necessity of a pressing medical procedure, for example, would require a shorter term of treatment than providing help about retirement issues. It is important to acknowledge that most older people do not enter therapy with the intention of changing their character structures or personalities, which makes a task-focused or problem-solving approach more practical than a strict psychoanalytic approach. It is important to clarify that a problem-solving orientation does not obviate the importance of forming an attachment with the patient or exploring the emotional and interpersonal implications of the individual's thoughts and behavior. The orientation is merely recommended as a practical framework for the patient-therapist interaction.

Choosing Psychotherapy

Treatment will vary according to the patient's functional age and the assessment of specific problems. The contract will be determined by these factors. The treatment must be tailored to the character structure of the client, as with any age cohort. In other words, a borderline character structure will require that the therapist place a great deal of emphasis upon creating a safe environment for the patient. There is also more of a need for setting limits with the borderline personality than with a more organized personality. If the patient is suffering from an organic disorder, then there are specific techniques that can be tried to improve cognitive functioning, such as sensory training, and reality orientation. If the patient has a well-organized personality and is not experiencing severe depression, anxiety, and/or guilt, attention may be focused on completion of tasks. Analysis of the individual's defenses or transference phenomena will take place within the framework of task completion. In other words, when anger toward the therapist surfaces as an obstacle to completion of the task, then the anger will become a focus for examination.

The major distinction between working with an older person rather than a younger individual is that the older person generally will not be interested in changing his or her personality. That is why the present model emphasizes the importance of establishing specificity of purpose and is task centered.

Another important feature of psychotherapy with the elderly is the need for the therapist to become involved in the life of the individual, coordinating different spheres of his or her activity. The therapist should be prepared to deal with families, doctors, lawyers, and social agencies. Case management is part of the treatment; this approach places the older client squarely at the center of the process, in contrast with other models, which view the client's family or else the system as the client. Here there is no such dilemma: the older person is the client. The goal is to mediate the exchange between the client and his or her informal and formal systems.

If, however, an adult child requests assistance in managing an aging parent, then the adult child is the client. The therapist, in this case, does not automatically assume responsibility for the treatment of the parent in addition to the child. Should this happen, there is potential for a conflict of interests, and, as with any age cohort, such potential outcomes should be carefully evaluated. If the conflict cannot be successfully mediated, the older person should be referred to another therapist.

Reminiscence—Life Review

Reminiscence, or "life review," is a technique that needs evaluation on a case-by-case basis. As with any other technique, its efficacy is situational. For some individuals the life review is helpful in fostering a sense of pride, self-acceptance, and greater self-esteem. For other, perhaps more fragile individuals, life review may be no more than "dredging up a painful past." Reminiscence has a specific place when counseling a memory-impaired individual. For this person life review can offer an escape from the frustrations of struggling with current events and perceptions. Many individuals enjoy providing a detailed personal and family history, and a type of life review is afforded by conducting a comprehensive intake interview. Reminiscence is often conducted in a group, so that, in addition to providing an opportunity for personal growth, it also encourages socialization and support.

Follow-up

An important component of counseling the elderly is coordinating other professional and informal services and providing "continuity-of-care" management. Case management is part of this job description. Even after the direct services to a client are terminated, or when acute therapy ends, the therapist remains an integral part of the individual's life. Monitoring the client's situation is essential; this involves everything from phone consultation with professionals to contacts with family members. Of all the professionals who work with the elderly, mental health practitioners have the greatest responsibility for conducting a comprehensive patient assessment and following up by addressing needs that have been identified; advising is, after all, intrinsic to the role.

Many factors have an impact on the mental health of an individual, including biological, medical, family, and institutional factors. For example, hearing impairment can lead to paranoia, a high fever or trauma to a delusional episode, financial or legal concerns to depression, and long-term care planning to family discord. It is incumbent upon the mental health professional to sort out the characterological influences from the social or medical factors affecting an older client's mental functioning. Differential diagnosis is crucial to ensuring proper treatment. The older person is subject to a greater risk of depression and involuntary polypharmacy than others, and, because of increasing frailty, is more likely to suffer family and institutional victimization. If one is dependent upon Social Security for one's livelihood, the government controls the purse strings. The connection between physical health and mental health is inextricable. A comprehensive assessment of the factors affecting the mental health of the individual is essential in treating mental disturbances.

64

REFERENCES

Belsky, J. K. (1984). *The psychology of aging.* Monterey, Calif.: Brooks/Cole.

Caine, E. D., J. M. Lyness, and D. A. King. (1993). Reconsidering depression in the elderly. *American Journal of Geriatric Psychiatry* 1, no. 1 (Winter): 4–20.

Greene, R. R. (1986). *Social work with the aged and their families.* New York: Walter de Gruyter.

Hendricks, J., and D. C. Hendricks. (1986). *Aging in mass society: Myths and realities.* Boston: Little, Brown.

Lamy, P. P. (1993). Understanding and managing Alzheimer's disease. *Pharmacy Times* (February): 95.

Travis, J. (1993). New piece in Alzheimer's puzzle. *Science* 261, 13 August, 828–29.

Weiner, M. A., A. J. Brok, and A. M. Snadowsky. (1987). *Working with the aged.* Norwalk, Conn.: Appleton-Century-Crofts.

Chapter 5

LEGAL DILEMMAS
Implications for Health and Social Functioning

Legal or financial concerns often serve as the catalyst for an older person's entry into the professional service arena. These concerns range from questions regarding applications for Social Security to eligibility for Medicaid, including the spending and transfer of assets or the need to plan for impending mental or physical incapacity. This chapter focuses on the legal dilemmas that typically confront aging people and the interplay of legal concerns with social or psychological concerns.

The role of the attorney in comprehensive screening is crucial. The attorney is a professional who most everyone goes to, at one time or another, for advice and counsel. Often investigation of legal issues causes a flood of practical and emotional concerns from the sick or aging client. Rather than cut off the flow of these concerns, a competent legal practitioner must be able to sort out their legal aspects from those related to health or spiritual matters. Many attorneys who specialize in elder law have developed collegial relationships with social workers or geriatric care managers to ensure comprehensive client service.

This chapter begins with a review of the legal services that older people typically need. These services include those related to planning for retirement, estate planning, and long-term care planning. In addition to those services involved with planning one's financial future, legal services tend to be grouped around health-related matters, such as the issuance of a living will or appointment of a health proxy. Laws pertaining to planning for incapacity and health care decision making are addressed. Protective service options are also addressed as appropriate. In addition, discharge planning laws and regulations serve as protections for individuals from unsafe hospital discharges or transfers and represent another focus of legal activity. It is important to acknowledge that there is some disparity in state laws governing health care, since states have a wide range of discretion in this area. The area of elder abuse represents another aspect of the attorney's concern. The services of an attorney cross-cut many legal specialties, including criminal law and constitutional law. For example, older people are often the targets of discrimination in employment and may seek legal recourse when confronted with unfair employment practices.

The chapter presents a description of each of the following legal services: retirement planning, estate planning, financial and social planning for incapacity, health care decision making, protecting against age discrimination, and preventing elder abuse. The implications of presenting legal issues for other areas of client functioning are identified to illustrate the importance of comprehensive assessments and multidisciplinary collaboration.

RETIREMENT PLANNING

The older client may seek the assistance of an attorney in filing an application for Social Security or Supplemental Security Income (SSI). The Social Security laws are complex; in general, however, the monthly amount received by the beneficiary is in direct proportion to the amount of time and money that a retired worker, and/or his or her spouse, has contributed to the system. With respect to Social Security individuals become eligible, at age sixty-two, to receive a permanently reduced benefit or, at age sixty-five, the full benefit allowance. Women who have not earned Social Security credits of their own are eligible to receive a percentage of their husbands' benefits. Generally, women, and primarily women of color, either receive a restricted allowance or Supplemental Security Income, a benefit that is available for the indigent. This phenomenon is a result of the sporadic or part-time employment history of women who are currently in the sixty-two-and-over age category.

It is not advisable for an individual to initiate financial planning on the verge of retirement. Most people maintain their general legal practitioner over the course of a lifetime. It is advisable, therefore, for a general legal practitioner to provide some guidance in financial matters early enough in the client's earning years to ensure the client's future security. Since many women are not in jobs that provide pensions, they are at greater risk all around. For example, not only are they likely to receive a smaller Social Security allowance than their male counterparts, but they are also less likely to have a retirement pension. It is very difficult to live on a Social Security allowance alone. There are many investment opportunities that are available to consumers, though a detailed discussion of them is beyond the scope of the present writing. A variety of tax-deferred annuities, mutual funds, and long-term savings bonds, however, offer conservative opportunities for investment. Most lawyers are able to refer clients for financial planning assistance, thus helping them avoid financial problems later in life.

Many older clients may not have planned effectively for retirement or may not have had certain investment opportunities available to them. They will need assistance in putting together a survival plan. This survival plan must include a consideration of "in-kind" benefits as well as supplementary monetary allowances. Subsidized housing or home share programs offer affordable housing options for people on limited budgets. Meal programs, such as Meals on Wheels, offer food subsidies to people in need, and senior centers provide lunch programs. There are many resources available for people in need, and an attorney must either be familiar with these services or be able to refer individuals to appropriate community agencies or private geriatric care managers for proper guidance.

ESTATE PLANNING

Elder lawyers often participate in the planning of clients' estates. In fact, the estate plan is considered to be the core of the legal consultation with the elderly (Freedman and WanderPolo 1993). Estate planning is a ripe area for comprehensive assessment and intervention. It is also fertile ground for family conflicts. Many attorneys have reported the reluctance of an older client to complete the estate plan. This reluctance may stem from the client's fear of mortality or, more likely, from family interference. It is easy to imagine the potential for intimidation in a situation in which the older person is dependent upon another's physical assistance.

The estate means more than money or assets to the elderly. It is an individual's legacy. The emotional connections are obvious. The estate plan may serve as an opportunity for the individual to come to terms with his or her own life and its impact on close family, friends, and community. It is obvious that a perceptive attorney should be on the alert for signs of emotional or spiritual unrest in the planning process (Fowler 1993).

PLANNING FOR INCAPACITY

Planning for incapacity incorporates many elements, including financial issues as well as continuity of care considerations. Lawyers not only plan estates but also frequently serve as the executor or trustee of a will. In these roles the attorney may be asked to assume certain fiduciary responsibilities and is then charged with investment duties (Fowler 1993). Similarly, an attorney can be charged with fiduciary responsibility for a trust fund created for a client who is at serious risk of becoming incapable of handling his or her own finances. The appointment of a trustee and the establishment of a trust fund is one means available to an individual for avoiding a court-ordered appointment of a conservator or adult guardian.

For the purposes of dealing with the Social Security Administration and similar state agencies, a competent individual also has the option of authorizing a representative payee to handle income and pay bills. An individual can also give a general power of attorney to another to handle a broad array of financial matters. Attorneys often fill these roles for their clients. Other service providers should be aware of the importance of addressing the need to plan financially for incapacity among their older clients and utilize the services of a legal expert. Lawyers should also be on the alert for signs of mental or physical change in older clients which signal the need for medical, social, or psychological intervention.

LONG-TERM CARE PLANNING

Planning for incapacity may include placement in an extended-care facility such as an adult home or a nursing home. This type of planning also includes a financial aspect, since long-term care is not covered by either Medicare, standard indemnity plans, or managed-care plans. Long-term care policies that presently exist should be seriously scrutinized (Kerr 1993). The premiums will probably outweigh any potential benefit unless the client has more than five hundred thousand dollars in cash assets.

One weakness in our present health delivery system is that the average individual must become impoverished in order to qualify for long-term care insurance under Medicaid. Most people can hardly afford to pay privately for nursing home care for more than a limited time period after their Medicare or private insurance benefits are exhausted. Some states, however, offer opportunities to protect assets by means of transfers, gifts, or the creation of special needs' trusts. In New York State the community spouse is offered some protection against impoverishment, while the institutionalized spouse is ensured eligibility for Medicaid.

Many factors have to be considered by aging couples. First, only 5 percent of those in the over-sixty-five age group presently are institutionalized in nursing homes. Twenty-five percent of those who are institutionalized are over age eighty-five. Most individuals will require some form of community health care in lieu of residential care. The rules in a particular state for eligibility for public assistance for home care should be carefully reviewed with a social worker and an attorney. Medicare and private insurance provide very restricted benefits. Consideration should be given to the way in which a couple's finances are organized—for example, in joint accounts and/or separate accounts or by individual and/or joint ownership of property.

PLACEMENT OPTIONS

Long-term care does not only mean nursing home care. Today there are many options for individuals which preclude the necessity of placement in a nursing home. Attorneys should be familiar with these alternative supportive living arrangements. Following is a list of extended care or supportive living alternatives and a brief description of each:

Homes for Adults

There are many types of homes for adults, including "family-like" residences, which provide homey environments, and institutional residences, which serve a greater number of people in a dormitory-type facility. These homes provide a variety of supports, including meals, personal care, medical supervision, and outreach to the community. Many of these homes are "for profit" and require private pay. Some homes will accept Social Security or SSI when the resident's personal resources are depleted.

Supportive Housing

Supportive housing options have evolved to allow older people to remain in the community and to live independently (Libby and Yates). These apartment buildings provide services ranging from social services to homemaking, housekeeping, and convenient neighborhood shopping. Many are run as not-for-profit entities and are subsidized. Many residences require private pay and are beyond what individuals on restricted incomes can afford. As with nursing home admissions, the more money one has, the greater the choice of housing opportunities. It is advisable to seek placement while one still has personal resources to offer upon admission. Some establishments want a family member to guarantee private payment, and this can create an obstacle or a family conflict. The use of an attorney to mediate can be very helpful in this situation.

Life Care Communities

Life care communities are comprehensive living arrangements that offer a range of social and health services. The great attraction of a life care community is that the resident is guaranteed a lifetime membership (Harvard Health Letter 1994). If the resident's health becomes seriously compromised, the community offers either skilled nursing on the premises or automatic transfer to a skilled nursing facility (SNF). These communities are run either by voluntary not-for-profit agencies or by proprietary organizations (for profit). A member must make a substantial financial investment, usually the purchase of a health care bond, which is redeemable by the heirs at the resident's death or transfer. It is important to evaluate the fiscal solvency of each community under consideration. An attorney, an accountant, or real estate expert can be useful in helping with the selection of such a living arrangement.

Nursing Homes

Nursing homes or skilled nursing facilities are a very restrictive placement option. In the 1980s nursing homes attempted to change their negative image as warehouses for the infirm to that of engaging residential homesteads. They attempted to attract highly functioning individuals who merely required limited personal support, such as meals, ambulatory assistance, and/or chore services. Today, because of concerns with cost containment, nursing homes have become the principal province of the most limited members of the community. No longer is there a distinction made between intermediary care and skilled nursing.

Most nursing home residents suffer at least some degree of cognitive impairment and are among the oldest and frailest members of the population. The current service continuum does not allow people to age to the point of disability in adult homes or supportive housing. Therefore, the move from one's home may involve two shifts and, consequently, two opportunities for trauma in an older person's life. The move to a nursing home generally is an alternative of least resort and, therefore, carries the weight of a "final sentence" for most people. If our health and social service system were less fragmented and homes for adults were legally and financially geared to provide increased supportive services, then these traumas could be avoided. To do this requires a change in the way services are insured and a restructuring of state Social Service and Health Departments.

Currently, there has been a substantial shift in service provision from the nursing home to the community and to homes for adults—without accompanying shifts in financing. The older individual is often caught up in these policy conflicts, and his or her movement in the system is fraught with difficulties. These difficulties usually drive the older person and his or her family members to an attorney's office.

It is not a good rule to wait until a crisis hits to seek legal assistance. Laws governing eligibility for public assistance require that applicants meet a financial means test. Transfers of assets have to be made according to certain legal criteria and within specific time frames in order for the elderly to qualify. The importance of recognizing failing mental or physical health and planning for incapacity is important from both a financial and a quality-of-life perspective. Each aspect should be given appropriate consideration.

QUALITY OF LIFE: LEGISLATION REGARDING HEALTH CARE DECISION MAKING

The issues surrounding legal aspects of health care decision making are extremely complex. The right to life, liberty, and the pursuit of happiness is espoused in the Declaration of Independence. The right to liberty serves as the basis of the right to self-determination, including the right to decide upon health care alternatives. The right of privacy and principles of due process are firmly and definitively supported in the Bill of Rights. The individual's right of consent to all medical procedures and plans regarding the course of care derives from these basic precepts.

The law is very clear with respect to the rights of a person of sound mind to direct the course of his or her health care. We run into some confusion with the rights of a person who is no longer capable of making his or her own decisions because of mental dysfunction or disability. In recent years, to avoid the necessity of a judge's ruling on every conflict regarding the course of a mentally incapable individual's treatment, most state's have enacted certain statutes detailing "advanced directives." Advanced directives range from statements of the individual's wishes regarding the right to refuse resuscitation to the contents of living wills and the appointment of health care agents. These laws allow the competent individual to make choices regarding the quality of life and/or the selection of a surrogate decision maker in the event of incapacity (Rowland 1992).

The "do not resuscitate" legislation generally involves the individual's wishes that cardiopulmonary resuscitation be withheld in certain situations. For example, a patient who has become unconscious may wish resuscitation to be withheld if he or she would be left in a "permanently vegetative state" if revived. The procedures surrounding administration of the law are also complex and may limit the scope of the directive's authority. In New York State, for example, the directive is effective only if a person is in an institution at the time of the medical emergency or in transport between institutions.

The health care proxy and living will are alternative methods for directing future medical intervention or nonintervention, in the event of a loss of mental capacity. The health care proxy allows the competent individual to select a surrogate, who is then entrusted with the individual's own power of decision making in health care matters. The living will is a written document that specifies treatment choices in particular medical situations. Since the medical profession is traditionally geared toward saving lives, the specificity and clarity of these directives is important in ensuring proper compliance.

Some states have one form of directive or the other. There is no universal policy governing the promulgation of advanced directives. The elder attorney is familiar with the nuances of the state legislation and can be effective in ensuring conformity with an elder client's wishes. Although the forms are drafted and can usually be prepared without the assistance of an attorney, consultation regarding the consequences of stating one's wishes is advisable.

CONSENT IN DISCHARGE PLANNING

The individual's right of consent is very central to laws of health care decision making. This right is not limited to treatment decisions. It also includes decisions having to do with continuity of care, planning, and discharge from a health facility. Lawyers must recognize that their legal responsibility to the older person requires an understanding of the policies of health agencies and institutions. Hospital discharge planning policies may challenge the individual's right of consent.

There is a simple principle that underlies hospital discharge policy: discharge patients as quickly as possible. This principle derives from the current system of hospital financing, or diagnostic-related group system. The DRG system is a prospective system of reimbursement in which hospitals are paid according to the diagnosis of a patient, regardless of the length of the patient's stay. Essentially, the quicker a patient is discharged, the sooner "the bed" (space) becomes available for another patient. The admission rate is directly related to the reimbursement rate, or, in other words, "the more patients that are admitted, the greater the total third-party reimbursement." This policy pressures hospitals to discharge patients. This affects patients with the most serious discharge issues, such as those requiring some sort of after-care.

The older patient is likely to require post-hospital care because of his or her frailty and the inherent complications of managing chronic diseases. Time is needed for equivalent planning. As a result of discharge pressures, patients are expected to leave acute hospitals as soon as medical clearance is provided. Although the hospital is required by law to see that a discharge plan is in place and to involve the patient and family in planning, the hospital's arrangement may not represent the patient's own interests. This statement is not meant as a condemnation of hospitals and hospital policies. In order to survive financially, institutions must operate in fiscally responsible ways. The statement is made to underscore the concept that patients have rights, and one of those rights is to refuse any discharge plan that is not acceptable. This right of refusal relates as emphatically to issues associated with discharge as to issues related to treatment.

An attorney generally can be effective in mediating between the needs of his or her client and the purposes of the hospital. In addition, in situations that require a more forceful stance, an attorney can be a useful patient advocate.

ETHICAL ASPECTS OF HEALTH CARE DECISIONS

The role of religious leaders and the centrality of spiritual concerns in the older person's life are explored in detail in the next chapter. There is a strong connection between law and ethics which is brought into extremely sharp focus in the area of health care decision making. This connection warrants special scrutiny and, thus, is elaborated in this section.

Decisions regarding treatment or care planning have more than a legal component. There is a distinctively spiritual aspect to decision making in this arena which highlights the close relationship of law, religion, and philosophy. The religious, metaphysical, or ethical leader is potentially an essential team member in health institutions. In the community practice field it is up to individual practitioners to make appropriate connections with professionals who can advise about ethical conflict and resolution. The astute attorney must be able to recognize ethical dilemmas at the root of a client's difficulty in reaching a health decision.

There are ethical aspects to decisions regarding everything from estate planning to planning for incapacity. In estate planning the client may be struggling with the fair appropriation of assets. In retirement planning husbands and wives may struggle with balancing self-interest with the interests of the spouse. Decisions regarding refusal of treatment or the withdrawal of life support have obvious ethical implications. For example, the decision to allow oneself to die requires an individual to accept the value of quality of life as being more important than mere survival. The law restricts certain choices, regardless of preference. For example, active euthanasia is prohibited throughout the nation, and poison cannot be administered or taken to expedite death. Judges in many jurisdictions have ruled, however, to permit the withdrawal of life support, including oxygen, food, and water. These decisions have been made on a case-by-case basis. There is as yet no legal statute governing the withdrawal of treatment.

The ethical arguments surrounding the "right to die" focus on the conflict between the individual's right of self-determination versus the individual's need to be "protected from him- or herself." Similarly, arguments regarding continuity of care planning highlight the conflict between individual autonomy and the need for protection. The law reflects these controversies. The lawyer's task in promoting his or her client's self-interest is not always clear. Many decisions imply the need for spiritual analysis, and coordination with the appropriate religious or ethical consultant is advisable.

AGE DISCRIMINATION IN THE WORKPLACE

Older people's vulnerability also extends into their work lives. There are many factors that impact upon the older person's employment experience, and age discrimination is one of them (Robinson et al. 1985). Furthermore, older people may require different accommodations and community supports in order to continue to work, such as lighting accommodations that serve to reduce glare or reliable transportation. Peters (1989) identifies discrimination as a major impediment to hiring the disabled individual. Older people may fall into this category because of the high incidence of chronic illness among the elderly. The widespread perception of age as an obstacle to employment can adversely influence an older person's motivation to seek employment, further compounding his or her difficulties (Nathanson and O'Rourke 1994).

There is some evidence to suggest that older people will become more desirable to employers in the future because of part-time employment trends and growth in the service sector of the economy (Personick, cited in Robinson et al. 1985). A projected reduced labor pool of younger workers can also help to explain this anticipated trend. Yet the current downsizing of industries in the United States serves as an additional threat to the older employee who may be viewed as obsolete. Consequently, older people's need for legal assistance may also stem from the fragility of their position in the job market.

ELDER ABUSE

Older people are easy targets for victimization. Elder abuse takes many forms. Many older people are benignly neglected by careless "caregivers." Others are physically abused. Some are financially and emotionally victimized and others sexually abused. The reasons for this abuse may vary, but there are some generalizations that can be made regarding its occurrence. Generally, older people are physically weaker than their victimizers. Often they are involved in a dependency relationship with the perpetrator of the abuse; many times the perpetrator is dependent upon the victim for financial or emotional support. The older person will probably be reluctant to tell of the abuse, most likely out of fear of retaliation or a reluctance to involve the authorities.

A lawyer may have to use his or her powers of discernment to identify abusive situations. It is, therefore, critical that attorneys take the time to get to know their older clients and make sure that they speak independently to older clients, regardless of the nature of the presenting problem. What may be presented by a son or daughter as a simple issue of arranging a financial transfer may turn out to be a matter of family coercion. The attorney should be on the lookout for signs of physical or mental abuse. If an older person hesitates to speak, this may be an indication of intimidation by family members.

Older people do not always know their rights. They also may not be aware of available protective services. A case in point is that of a woman who, after fifty years of marriage, decided she wanted to leave her husband. She was sent to a psychiatrist, who wisely sent her to an attorney. The family wanted her to be medicated. She wanted to be out of the marriage. She was empowered by the knowledge that she could leave her husband and have financial independence. The fact that she chose to stay with him is inconsequential. That she now has a sense of independence is of monumental significance.

Sometimes an older person will resist intervention because the alternatives seem worse than the present reality. The system may not provide a clearly reasonable option. Most states do not have mandatory reporting laws for elder abuse. Such laws are considered by many to deprive the older person of his or her right of self-determination. As already stated, it is also extremely difficult to come up with an appropriate plan for dealing with elder abuse, given the lack of subsidized living arrangements and the restrictions on nursing home admission. These potential snags must be unraveled to reveal the benefits of protection to the older person. It is the authors' belief that, in areas related to abuse or potential abuse, it is generally better for a professional to err on the side of commission rather than omission; in other words, it is better to do too much than too little.

Careful planning and the use of collateral resources, such as the services of a geriatric care manager or social worker, can very often be effective in liberating a person from a harmful situation. Furthermore, ultimately, it is primarily the older person's choice to decide how to proceed in a given situation. It is important to remember, even in situations in which the older person is suffering from some form of cognitive impairment, that, legally, a person is considered to be competent unless deemed incompetent in a court of law. If the person's competency is at issue, than the attorney must consider filing for guardianship or the appropriate protective service option. This mandate also applies in matters related to estate or retirement planning or planning for incapacity.

IMPLICATIONS OF LEGAL DILEMMAS

The relationship of the attorney's role to other practitioners is investigated in detail in chapter 9. The present discussion focuses on the implications of legal problems for other areas of client functioning.

The emotional implications of legal decisions are legion. Estate planning, for example, requires an individual to confront his or her own mortality. This process can be tantamount to buying a burial plot or planning one's own funeral. Retirement also represents intense loss for many people, second only to losing one's mate. It is not difficult to imagine the overwhelming anxiety that can infuse the process of planning for this eventuality. Consider the depth of the feelings associated with recognition of impending physical or mental frailty. As the threat of loss looms larger, older people are likely to cling more tightly to its fleeting vestiges.

Elder lawyers deal with sickness, death, and bereavement; it is the nature of the job. Consequently, it is imperative that lawyers be attuned to all of the mental and physical ramifications of their clients' conflicts. The effects of stress or prolonged grieving can undermine an individual's health and functioning and mask other chronic mental problems as well. Spiritual or ethical uncertainties play havoc with the soul. Just as lawyers must be aware of the implications of legal presenting problems for other areas of client functioning, it is equally important that other human service providers be aware of the association between law and other aspects of client functioning, including spiritual ones.

Legal issues that typically face the aging individual run the gamut from those related to matters of financial management to those associated with continuity of care management. The older person must plan for retirement in order to ensure financial independence. With people living longer and being healthier, many do not want to, or cannot afford to, prepare for an early retirement. Yet the system does not currently support these shifts in life expectancy and job prospects. The older person may need help with problems of living and working as well as with those related to loss and illness. The lawyer will be confronted with a range of concerns. Among these are the need to plan for a client's incapacity, the need to execute a will, and the need to secure benefits for the client. Each of these concerns is laden with emotional and spiritual conflicts that are best evaluated by a psychotherapist or member of the clergy.

The advantage to coordinating with other service providers does not only fall to the client. The lawyer benefits as well. Proper coordination of services liberates the attorney to do what he or she is trained to do, with a clear understanding of what will better ensure a successful outcome. Conversely, each member of the multidisciplinary network benefits from appropriate coordination with the legal expert.

REFERENCES

Fowler, J. (1993). Investing funds of an estate: The attorney's responsibilities. Paper presented at New York County Lawyer's Association, New York.

Freedman, R., and M. WanderPolo. (1993). Putting it all together: Estate planning for the elderly client. *New York State Bar Journal* 65, no. 6 (September–October): 40–43.

Kerr, P. (1993). Elderly care: The insurer's role. *New York Times,* 15 March.

Libby, J., and B. Yates, eds. N.d. *Housing guide for senior citizens.* New York: Office of Public Information.

Nathanson, I., and K. O'Rourke. (1994). The job interests of older workers in a suburban employment training program. *Journal of Gerontological Social Work* 21 (Summer): 3–4.

Peters, J. E. (1989). How to bridge the hiring gap. *Personnel Administrator* (October): 76–85.

Retirement living—picking a place. (1994). *Harvard Health Letter* (January): 9.

Robinson, P. K., S. Coberly, and C. E. Paul. (1985). Work and retirement. In *Handbook of aging and the social sciences,* ed. R. Binstock and E. Shanas, 503–27. New York: Van Nostrand Reinhold.

Rowland, M. (1992). Planning for the end of life. *New York Times,* 22 March.

Chapter 6

RELIGIOSITY, SPIRITUALITY, AND ETHICAL ISSUES
Including Religious Organizations in the Service Network

This chapter explores the role of religion, religious leaders, and religious organizations in the lives of older adults. The integration of religious organizations with community organizations can offer an opportunity to fill a gap created by national, state, and local government efforts in the delivery of human services. The authors explain how religious leaders can be a part of the multidisciplinary community team that enhances the lives of older adults.

It is demonstrated in the literature that religion plays a major role in the life of older persons. The church, synagogue, or other place of worship remains one of the most important organizations in an older person's life (Tobin et al. 1985). Religion is important in the lives of Americans generally (Taylor 1993), and its presence in one's life has been positively related to overall satisfaction (Tobin 1985). Yet there is still debate about the contribution religion makes to the life satisfaction of older adults. Moberg (1975) found that older persons are members of religious organizations more than of any of the other types of voluntary social organizations combined. Some writers suggest that religion assumes a more prominent place in the lives of older adults due to the onset of chronic health problems, which can heighten their fears as well as their desire to find comfort, and the realization of their own mortality (Taylor 1993). Spirituality has been related to well-being among older adults (Hooyman and Kiyak 1993).

The role of religious organizations and their impact upon the lives of people have changed throughout history. Religious organizations, historically, have served many social functions, such as providing food to the poor, helping families, and housing the sick, the old, and the disabled. The role of the religious

79

organization changed dramatically after the Reformation, when the separation of church and state became a central issue for governments and churches. The influence of churches upon governing rulers during the Middle Ages led to the persecution of innocent victims in the name of religion. In the period following the Middle Ages colonization created countries that demanded freedom of religion and freedom from persecution due to one's religious affiliation. The separation of church and state was a major issue in America in colonial times. Colonial America insisted on a government that was free from specific religious ties. Americans continue this tradition into the twentieth century, remaining dedicated to the policy of separation of church and state, and it is in this context that churches have abandoned many of their traditional social functions. Some of the social services previously provided by religious organizations have become the responsibilities of governments. Yet government is no longer able to fill the needs for social assistance that each community demands.

Historically, religious leaders have held teaching and leadership roles. In the past religious persons were spiritual leaders who offered guidance for the day-to-day activities of one's life. Ethical issues were decided by spiritual leaders, and spirituality was deeply involved in all aspects of life. The English painter Thomas Cole's early-nineteenth-century series *Journey of Life* depicts each of life's stages, from birth, youth, middle age, through old age, as directed by an angel of God. Religion was deeply intertwined with life and death.

THE GRAYING OF RELIGIOUS ORGANIZATIONS

The population of Americans over sixty-five is 13 percent, or thirty-one million. It is obvious that, as Americans are aging, members of churches are aging also.

In 1991 the U.S. Census Bureau report for religious preference in the United States was 56 percent Protestant, 25 percent Catholic, 2 percent Jewish, 6 percent "Other," and 11 percent "None." Sixty-eight percent of the population belonged to a religious organization. In 1991, 76 percent of this group were over fifty years of age (U.S. Bureau of the Census 1993). Currently, some denominations are assessing the percentage of older persons in their own congregations. The Presbyterian churches report that over 55 percent of their congregations are over fifty years of age (Morgan 1994). The Catholic churches are reporting aging congregations as well as aging priests (Lewis 1994). The Catholic church has over twenty thousand parishes throughout the United States. It appears that members of the Catholic parishes are aging more quickly than the population in general. In a study by Fordham University's Third Age Center the preliminary report found that the percentage of church members over the age of sixty-five years was greater than the national average (Lewis 1994). Catholic parishes

80

reported at least 26 percent of their members to be over sixty-five years.

Studies based on data from the National Survey of Black Americans indicate a high degree of religious commitment among older black adults (Taylor 1993). Older black adults report that they attend church regularly, feel that it is very important in their lives, and are likely to be active church members. Many social and political functions have been attributed to the church in the African-American community. Some scholars suggest that during slavery the church functioned as an agency of social control (Smith 1993). During the civil rights era the church served as an arena for political functions. Today the African-American church may even function as a social service agency. A study by Glover and Sinkler-Parker (1994) found that some of the African-American churches offer specific social services, such as transportation to medical appointments and home-cooked meals. Another study found that over 50 percent of church leaders were over fifty years old and that congregations reported from 40 to 70 percent of their members to be over sixty-five (Tirrito and Euster 1993).

It is necessary with an aging population to reexamine the role of religious organizations and religious leaders and their influence on the lives of older adults. In this book the authors contend that a new perspective is needed to link churches, synagogues, and other places of worship and religious leaders with their congregants. Older adults especially can benefit from this linkage. The domain of religious organizations needs to expand once again to incorporate social functions and teaching functions. The role of spiritual leadership is very important. The role of spiritual comforter is absolutely essential, yet religious leaders and religious organizations can do more than provide comfort and spiritual leadership. It is necessary for churches and synagogues to work collaboratively with community professionals to enhance the well-being of older adults. This chapter explores these issues and offers recommendations for religious leaders and religious organizations to consider in expanding their roles and responsibilities in an effort to help older adults.

As is suggested in the following story, we all travel the same road.

In the last century an American tourist visited the renowned Polish Rabbi Hofetz Chaim. The tourist was amazed to find the Rabbi's home only a simple room, filled with books, a table, and a bench.

"Rabbi," he asked. "Where is your furniture?"

"Where is yours?" asked the Rabbi.

"Mine?" asked the puzzled American. "But I'm only a visitor here. I'm only passing through."

"So am I," replied the Rabbi.

(Thorsen and Cook, quoted in Morgan 1990)

RELIGIOSITY AND OLDER ADULTS

It is necessary to distinguish between religiosity and spirituality. Religiosity refers to attendance at religious functions. Churches, synagogues, and other places of worship are very important to older adults, given that four out of five older adults (86 percent) believe in the existence of God. Three out of four of those age sixty and over report that religion is important in their lives. Four out of five of those over sixty-five attend a church, synagogue, or other place of worship regularly. The evidence suggests that people maintain their religious beliefs throughout their lives and those in the current cohort of elderly persons have been religious throughout their lives and continue to be so as they age (Tobin et al. 1986).

Attendance at a church, synagogue, or other place of worship is found to be lowest among those in their thirties, peaks in the late fifties and early sixties (60 percent of this age group attend religious services), and declines in the late sixties and early seventies. Yet this latter group still exceeds any other age group with over 50 percent of its members attending religious services. In addition, those in the over-sixty-five-year-old group are the most likely to be affiliated with religious groups or fraternal associations. Declines in attendance at formal services after age seventy may be attributed to health problems or transportation difficulties among the elderly, or perhaps churches and synagogues are not age conscious and do not offer opportunities for older members to participate in service activities.

Religion appears to be more important to older adults than to younger people. This may be true, however, of a particular cohort of older adults whose members also valued religion when they were younger. Religious beliefs must be separated from formal religious activities or church attendance. After age sixty religious beliefs tend to flourish (Hooyman and Kiyak 1993).

Ethnic and gender differences have been found in studies of religious activities. African-American older adults have been found to be more actively involved and have high rates of church membership. Both sexes indicate that religion is related to their well-being and life satisfaction (Hooyman and Kiyak 1993). For African-American older adults the church provides social services, counseling, and transportation. A profile of religious involvement found that older black adults have a higher probability of being religiously affiliated, of having attended religious services as an adult, and of being a church member. One major indicator of the spiritual and social importance of religion is the frequency of participation in religious services. In one study three out of four respondents indicated that they are official members of a church (Taylor 1993).

82

Mexican-American older adults were found to be more religious than white older adults, as measured by church attendance and self-rated religiousness and the frequency of private prayer. These three factors have been related to life satisfaction (Hooyman and Kiyak 1993).

RELIGION AND WELL-BEING

Studies have indicated that religiosity (defined as religious activities) is correlated positively with the well-being of older persons. Religious activities have been found to be associated positively with happiness and high morale. In some individuals age seventy-five and over religion was second to health in terms of maintaining morale (Hooyman and Kiyak 1993). The studies are not clear about whether the benefits of religion come from the meaning it gives to life or the social interaction it provides.

Spiritual well-being is called the affirmation of life (Tobin, Ellor, and Anderson-Ray 1986). Well-being is equated with a wholeness of life and with physical, psychological, and social good health. One's spiritual well-being cannot be separated from his or her physical or psychological well-being. Life satisfaction has been examined and studied by measuring a person's sense of well-being. The relationship between a sense of well-being and satisfaction with one's life, or happiness, has been found to be correlated positively (Neugarten 1977).

Yet spiritual well-being is defined by the National Interfaith Coalition as "the affirmation of life in a relationship with God, self, community and environment that nurtures and celebrates wholeness" (Tobin, Ellor, and Anderson-Ray 1986).From this perspective people can be spiritual without being religious in the sense of belonging to an organized religion (Hooyman and Kiyak 1993). Spiritual well-being has been associated with mental health, self-esteem, and social skills. The spiritual dimensions of health have been examined, and some practitioners view spiritual well-being as very important to an older person's physical and mental health. Health assessment tools are beginning to include questions about the individual's spiritual attitudes. Proponents of this approach advocate training for providers to include spiritual well-being in geriatric assessments.

The strength of religious affiliation of older adults has only recently been recognized as an influential force that can be used positively to enhance their well-being. Morgan in his book of readings *No Wrinkles on the Soul* (1990) presents a series of prayers and meditations for older adults. He discusses the importance of spirituality and the church in helping older adults meet the challenges of a "third age." Morgan is an ordained Presbyterian minister who is the author of several books about religion. He is concerned about the lack of ministries available to older adults. He suggests that methods be explored which will enhance the role and functions of religious leaders in the development of older-adult ministries. Religious leaders have not yet tapped their potential for providing spiritual and social assistance to older adults faced with many losses and impending death.

RELIGIOUS ORGANIZATIONS AS UNTAPPED RESOURCES

Nationally, there is recognition that religious organizations are untapped resources for future social services for older adults (Lewis 1993). Organized religion has concentrated its outreach programs on youths and families. Most churches develop youth ministries and try to increase the number of families and children in their congregations. Programs are directed at families with young children, and teens. Recently, churches, synagogues, and other places of worship have come to recognize the need to develop ministries specifically for older members. Church programs for older adults have seen a substantial growth at the national and local levels. Some services being offered are counseling, adult day care, in-home services, nutrition services, retirement training, and transportation. Socializing functions such as trips and bingo games are no longer adequate. Religious organizations can do more.

It is well established in the literature that older adults generally do not utilize the services of mental health clinics (Turner 1992). Because of the stigma attached to government programs, older adults are reluctant to use these services, even when they are available in communities. Religious organizations can help; social services offered by churches, synagogues, and other places of worship do not have a stigma attached to them. Thus, for example, attending a support group for newly bereaved men is more acceptable for many older people if group meetings are sponsored by the church or synagogue than by a local mental health clinic. An older adult who is severely depressed may be reluctant to seek treatment at a local mental health clinic but may accept treatment from a mental health therapist who is affiliated with his or her church or synagogue.

NEW OPPORTUNITIES

Hospice care was originally a religious service, the word *hospice* referring to offering hospitality or assistance to those in need. Religious organizations recognized their duty to help society's less fortunate members. In England the roots of the hospice movement began with St. Christopher's Home in London.

St. Christopher's is a place where the terminally ill can come to die in dignity and without pain. The hospice movement in this country began in 1973, when two hospices were built, one in California and one in Connecticut. In the 1980s hospice became medically linked with Medicare and Medicaid reimbursement. In the late 1980s and the 1990s the hospice movement expanded to include home-based service for the terminally ill. Currently, hospice programs are affiliated with hospitals and with home care programs. The underutilization of the hospice program is a source of concern. It is possible, however, that the medicalization of the hospice program has not served its best interests; the loss of religious affiliation and spirituality has been detrimental to the hospice movement. Dying is a spiritual process as well as a physical process. Meeting one's spiritual needs at the last stage of life is the domain of religion, not medicine.

Religious organizations can help to fill the gaps in social services which government has been unable to fill. There are numerous opportunities to provide programs and services that benefit older adults. Churches, synagogues, and other religious organizations are becoming aware that ministry to older adults must involve more than has been offered in the past (Lewis 1994). There are many needed programs that are not being adequately handled by social service agencies, such as Meals on Wheels, respite programs, volunteer chore programs, mental health screening, legal and financial planning, retirement planning, and support groups for families and for adult children. Social service agencies alone cannot meet the demands for these services. Churches can help. One elderly parishioner writes about her church: "My church is not fulfilling this need, but I have found some senior centers that are church sponsored and are an alternative for activities and programs for those fifty-five and older. I believe that churches should recognize and support programs for older adults." Another church member wrote: "Older members need rides; please help."

The Fordham University study completed by the Third Age Center made several recommendations to improve services for the elderly provided by religious organizations (Lewis 1993). The study was undertaken to examine how religious organizations could reach frail elderly in their homes. It initiated a program in which twenty-five selected coalitions of major congregations were awarded fifty thousand dollars a year for three years to identify frail people in their homes and to recruit and train volunteers to assist them. Data collection began in 1984 and continued until 1986. Some of the recommendations from this study were:

—The National Conference of Catholic Bishops should develop a pastoral on growing old in the community of faith. This document should articulate a series of principles and pastoral suggestions to give impetus to program-

ming in the nearly twenty thousand parishes in the United States.
—Each diocese should include an aging agenda item in its planning process.
   It should develop an ad hoc or ongoing work group to identify those
   opportunities for ministry of and to older persons.
—The church should encourage training of persons in aging ministry.
—Communities should look to parishes and diocesan leadership as integral to
   their efforts to serve older persons.
—The "aging network" under the leadership of the Administration on Aging,
   State Units on Aging, the National Association of State Units on Aging,
   and National Association of Areawide Agencies on Aging should initiate
   action to include parishes as a means of serving older persons.
—Formal social agencies, particularly hospitals, nursing homes, home care
   agencies and public social service agencies, should develop ongoing
   relationships with churches and synagogues. (Lewis 1993, 27).

   The conclusions from this study can be generalized to religious organizations
nationally, as follows:

—Churches and synagogues can develop many services and activities for
frail older persons.
—On the whole, they have done relatively little for older congregants generally and less for the frail.
—Generally, churches and synagogues lack a vision of service to older persons.
—While religious culture, ideology and history may influence the sense of
mission of local congregations, it seems that programmatic decisions are
influenced by local circumstances. Churches and synagogues have many
older congregants. They are integral to the ordinary life of the church and
synagogue.
—Older congregants tend to be taken for granted.
—Churches and synagogues can both find and gain access to frail, older
persons.
—Churches and synagogues are able to recruit, motivate and sustain volunteers.
—Churches and synagogues can make connections between those in need
and those ready to volunteer. However, it is unlikely they will be able to
generate substantial personal care services.
—Churches and synagogues are able to generate substantial human support
for frail persons with attendant services such as modest home repair, transportation, reassurance and socialization.

—While congregational services are unlikely to delay institutionalization directly, they may help indirectly by relieving the burden on the primary caregiver. (Lewis 1993, 28)

The recommendations and conclusions from this study should be implemented by religious organizations nationwide to enhance the well-being of older adults. Older adults have long been neglected by the type of organization they value most and to which many over the life span have contributed both financially and emotionally.

RELIGIOUS GERONTOLOGY'S GROWTH

Recently, aging studies have developed new interests in religion and gerontology. New journals such as the *Journal of Religion and Aging* and the *Journal of Religious Gerontology* offer articles that cover many areas of spirituality as well as articles that describe specific programs for elderly congregants. The focus of religious gerontology has been expanded in order to explore more than the spiritual well-being of older adults. It includes how religious organizations can improve their ministries to a heterogeneous group of aging congregants.

In addition, schools of theology have begun to acknowledge the graying of their churches and have included, in their curricula, courses with material on aging. A study by the Association for Gerontology in Higher Education found that schools of theology had increased the number of courses offered in courses related to the aging process (Payne and Brewer 1989).

Although increasing attention is being given to religious gerontology by churches, synagogues, and other religious organizations, one study found that current religious leaders have not had training in aging issues and were not interested in formal training courses. Thus, although we can expect future religious leaders to have some training, most of them today are not trained and, in fact, expressed an awareness that they were inadequately prepared to deal with issues affecting older members; nevertheless, they were not interested in acquiring more formal training (Tirrito and Euster 1993).

ENHANCING THE ROLE AND FUNCTIONS
OF RELIGIOUS LEADERS

The role and functions of religious leaders and religious organizations must be reexamined. What should, and can, they do to provide social services to their congregants? What teaching and leadership roles can they assume? Is it the religious organization's responsibility to provide these social services? Was it not promised in the Bible: "Even to your old age and gray hairs, I am he, I am he who will sustain you. I have made you and I will carry you: I will sustain you and I will rescue you" (Isa. 46:4 [New International Version])?

The activities of the clergy tend to center around problems. A spiritual leader is often the first person a family or individual turns to when confronted by crisis. The priest is called to administer the last rites at the time of impending death. The minister is called upon in times of serious illness. The rabbi is called upon to help with a decision to place a family member in a nursing home. The family who is faced with an ethical decision about whether or not life support systems should be maintained for a family member will often consult its spiritual leader for advice. An individual who is facing a painful death and prays for death to come needs comfort. Helping family members deal with suicide often becomes a religious leader's task. A spouse whose partner has Alzheimer's disease needs support. A parent whose adult child has AIDS needs consolation. An older person whose adult child is abusing or neglecting him or her may confide in the spiritual leader rather than report the problem to police or social agencies. Changes in the physical and mental condition of older adults can be detected by church leaders. The physical and emotional frailty of an older member can also be identified by other congregants in its early stages.

Who will provide the counsel needed in "right to die" issues? Medical advances have created a need for us to make "end-of-life" choices. Currently medical personnel are making these decisions rather than spiritual leaders. In times past a person who could not breathe would die. Today respirators, tube feeders, and hydration devices can help sustain life for years. Medical professionals and, most recently, the courts continue to make decisions about ending or prolonging life. As the timing of death has come later and later in life, ethical issues have grown up around end-of-life decisions. Should not this be the domain of religious leaders?

Is it enough for religious leaders to offer support and spiritual guidance in times of illness or impending death? Or should religious leaders provide other services? If so, which ones?

"Gatekeepers" (nontraditional sources of referral and information), direct services by volunteer members, counseling, and support groups are just some of the services that religious leaders and religious organizations can provide. The breadth of the list is determined by the willingness and concern of the leaders of these organizations, but in any case the first step is knowledge. Knowledge is necessary to understand the needs of the members of a religious community. The diversity of the elderly population and the diversity of religious organizations within various communities demand unique programs for each community. A sharing of knowledge—about services and programs that are effective—is simply a matter of communication between religious organizations and their members. Annual meetings are often the sites of much shared knowledge. The knowledge of ministries to older adults can be shared at these meetings. Moberg (1975) found that one-day conferences were excellent vehicles for imparting gerontological information to religious leaders.

Prior to this step, however, it is necessary to develop expertise and knowledge among religious leaders. As mentioned, most religious leaders today did not have the benefit of having material on aging during their early studies. Theological schools and seminaries have been very slow to recognize the need to teach aging content in their curricula. A survey of 202 evangelical churches chosen at random from across the country showed that 54 percent did not have a ministry to older adults, and 67 percent had only one activity per month for older people (Beal 1982). In another national study, sponsored by the Association for Gerontology in Higher Education, Payne and Brewer (1989) examined accredited seminaries in the United States to determine the status of gerontology in theological education. Their study found that, recently, there was significant attention being paid on the part of many seminaries to include gerontological material in their curricula.

Ministries to older adults are created by religious leaders who are knowledgeable about aging and interested in older adults (Moberg 1975). For successful ministries to older adults it is essential for the minister, priest, or rabbi to examine his or her attitudes toward aging to understand the differences between pathological and normal aging, to recognize mental health problems, to have adequate knowledge about legal issues confronting older adults, to be aware of the impact of health issues upon older persons, and to appreciate the diversity in the aging population.

COLLABORATION AMONG PUBLIC AGENCIES AND RELIGIOUS ORGANIZATIONS

How can religious organizations collaborate with public agencies to enhance the well-being of today's older adults and tomorrow's older adults? The leadership and teaching role has been largely neglected by religious leaders. There is an opportunity at this time to recapture the importance of the teaching function and leadership that spiritual leaders once demonstrated. In our society we are plagued with many unanswered ethical dilemmas. Medical technology has advanced so rapidly that we have not had time to address all the questions it has raised. At a recent church service a priest said that he believes in the promotion of life, not in the promotion of death. This is a dilemma in an aging society whose technology has been geared toward denying death.

Did God plan for us to interfere with death? Did God plan for us to intubate a ninety-five-year-old patient for several months to prevent the person from dying? Did God plan for a one-hundred-year-old comatose woman to spend two years in a hospital bed connected to feeding and breathing tubes? Did God plan for us to keep people alive in a comatose state? Does God want us to keep death away? These are some of the questions that spiritual leaders need to explore and enlighten us about.

Moody (1994) has posed some provocative ethical questions for our society:

1. Why do we grow old?
2. Should we ration health care on the grounds of age?
3. Should people have the choice to end their lives?
4. Should families provide for their own?
5. Does old age have meaning?

All of these questions need answers. Most important, we must explore the meaning of old age. Cole (1992), among others, has suggested that old age must have meaning, that there is a reason for aging. Why do we live to be eighty or ninety years old? Do we age so that we can give back to society our knowledge and wisdom? Do we age in order to give to younger persons an appreciation of life?

We are born to grow and develop. We reach adulthood and produce new generations, and we create a world for new generations to live in. But why do we age? What is the purpose of growing old? In trying to answer these questions—specifically, "Does old age have meaning?"—Moody offers a quote by Carl Jung: "A human being would certainly not grow to be seventy or eighty years old if this longevity had no meaning for the species. The afternoon of human life must also have a significance of its own and cannot be merely a pitiful appendage to life's morning" (Moody 1994, 395).

Spiritual leaders can and should help to answer these questions. Historically, Judaism has looked to the learned rabbi to answer profound questions. We need to look once again to religious leaders to help us find answers to some of the profound ethical dilemmas we have created in modern society. We have been successful in creating old age; now we must find its meaning.

Difficult decisions need to be made. Shall we legalize assisted suicide? Shall we consider voluntary euthanasia? In an aging society long life is a blessing for some, yet for others death is a welcome relief. Who should help resolve these issues? We believe that religious organizations can collaborate with public agencies to find answers to some of society's dilemmas and can help to develop appropriate policies. The contributions that religious leaders can make has not yet been tapped by policy makers.

COLLABORATION AMONG RELIGIOUS LEADERS AND COMMUNITY PROFESSIONALS

How can religious leaders collaborate with other professionals in the community to meet the needs of older adults? Religious leaders are usually well aware of the psychosocial problems of the members of their congregations. As one minister said, "When I look at my congregation on Sunday, I am sad to look at each face and think about the difficulties each person is dealing with in their lives." The problems of alcoholism, drug abuse, elder abuse, proper care, depression, and mental illness are among the issues that religious leaders are often asked to deal with in their organizations. For example, an older adult and his or her family members may seek counseling from a respected member of the clergy prior to considering formal therapy; often the religious leader is untrained to deal with such issues, especially in the case of older adults.

We believe that the spiritual leader of older adults can be an effective resource in assessment and referral to appropriate community professionals. It is not to be expected that the religious person take on the role of therapist or psychiatrist. It is suggested that the religious leader be prepared to assess the congregant's situation and appropriately refer the congregant to the community practitioner most qualified to deal with the problem. The religious leader must have gerontological knowledge to assess accurately the older person's situation.

CASE EXAMPLE

Barbara Allen tells her rabbi that her eighty-six-year-old mother is very difficult to live with. She explains that mom has been living with her for the past two years, after having moved from Chicago, where she lived until Dad died. Mom is unable to sleep, walks around the house most of the night, forgets to take her medicine, loses her dentures, and cries frequently. Other times Mom is angry, hostile, and unappreciative. Sometimes she is verbally abusive to her grandchildren. Barbara Allen's husband is losing his patience and becoming more and more angry at Mom. The children, age twenty and twenty-three, are ignoring her and spending less and less time talking to her and visiting her. This tends to make her more upset and tearful.

Mom refuses to attend the local senior center. She attends synagogue but will not participate in any other synagogue-related activities. There are no older women in the immediate neighborhood. Since Barbara Allen works during the day, Mom is home alone each day. In the evenings Mom wants to socialize, while Barbara would like some private and quiet time. Barbara is tearful and unhappy most of the time. She is not functionally well at her job. She frequently has to leave work early because her mother calls her with a crisis. Her employer noticed the change in her work and told her she needed to resolve her situation or her job would be at risk. Her husband wants her mother to live somewhere else. Barbara is feeling guilty and angry and shares these problems with her rabbi.

The religious leader can assess the situation and then make appropriate referrals to professional practitioners in the community. It seems that Mom would benefit from the evaluation of a geriatric psychiatrist, a physical examination from a geriatrician, and the help of a social worker who can seek out support groups in the community or alternate housing arrangements. In addition, Barbara Allen would benefit from a caregivers' support group.

Another example in which the religious leader can play a pivotal role involves a daughter who confides in the priest that her mother seems to be drinking excessively.

CASE EXAMPLE

Phyliss M., age seventy, has been widowed for two years. She has three sons and one daughter. After her husband died Phyliss M. came to live in the same community as her daughter. The other children live in New York, Atlanta, and Charleston. She has been in good health and is involved in church activities. She has some friends and socializes with them occasionally. Her daughter has noted, however, that, when she speaks to her mother in the evenings, her mother seems to have slurred speech and is not always coherent. The daughter has been concerned that her mother might be developing some physical or mental problem such as Alzheimer's disease. When she visits her mother unexpectedly, she finds empty bottles of wine and sherry. Her mother has explained that she drinks wine with dinner and sherry each evening to help her sleep. Phyliss M. has no previous history of alcohol abuse. Her daughter has discussed the issue of excessive alcohol use with her mother, who denies any abuse. Phyliss M. also denies having any other problems. Her daughter has discussed the matter with her brothers and sisters, who had not seen a problem with their mother having wine and sherry if it helps her and makes her sleep.

The religious leader can play an important role in this situation. The family has not previously been involved with social services agencies and will not consider referral to a mental health clinic for alcohol abuse treatment. Despite the trend toward less use of alcohol by all adults, many older adults drink alcohol, and some experience significant physical, social, emotional, and financial problems that are alcohol related. The incidence of late-life alcohol abuse was found to be significant in those age sixty-five to seventy-four and those age forty-five to fifty-four. A New York City study determined that older men who have lost their spouses are at greatest risk for alcohol-related problems than those who have not. Another study found that alcohol-related problems are an issue for women also (Farkas 1992).

This problem of alcohol abuse among older adults is neither widely recognized nor widely treated. Thus, a priest can act as a referral source to a community geropsychotherapist who is trained to deal with issues relating to alcohol abuse in older adults. The multidisciplinary community team effort would be very valuable in this situation and would provide the services needed by this family.

It is well known in the literature that elderly men are more likely to commit suicide than any other age group in the United States (Kaplan, Adamek, and Johnson 1994). In addition, the rate of suicide increased between 1979 and 1988. Religious leaders can play a pivotal role in identifying men who are at risk of suicide and referring these people to community professionals who can help them resolve some of their concerns.

What needs to be done? First, religious leaders must be aware of the dominant roles that they can play in the lives of their congregations, especially the lives of older adults. Second, religious leaders must be trained in gerontology to understand the biological, psychological, and social processes of aging. Third, religious leaders must develop within their churches, synagogues, and other places of worship programs and services for older adults. The material in this book will prove to be a useful tool in involving religious leaders in the community as part of a multidisciplinary team effort that is needed to enhance the well-being of older adults.

REFERENCES

Beal, D. P. (1982). Effective church ministry with older adults. *Journal of Christian Education* 3, no. 1: 5–17.

Carlson, R. W. (1985). The Episcopal seminaries and aging. *Journal of Religion and Aging* 1, no. 3: 1–11.

Cole, T. R. (1992). *The journey of life: A cultural history of aging in America.* New York: Cambridge University Press.

Glover, S., and C. Sinkler-Parker. (1994). A study of African-American churches and their services for older adults. Paper presented at the

National Council on Aging conference, Washington, D.C., May.

Hooyman, N., and H. A. Kiyak. (1993). *Social gerontology,* 3d ed. Boston: Allyn and Bacon.

Jackson, J., L. Chatters, and R. Taylor. (1993). *Aging in black America.* Beverly Hills, Calif.: Sage.

Kaplan, M. S., M. E. Adamek, and S. Johnson. (1994). Trends in firearm suicide among older American males. *Gerontologist* 34, no.1: 59–66.

Lewis, M. A. (1994). *Religious congregations and the informal supports of the frail elderly: Project summary.* New York: Fordham University.

Moberg, D. O. (1975). Needs felt by the clergy for ministries to the aging. *Gerontologist* 15, no. 2: 170–75.

Moody, H. R. (1994). *Aging concepts and controversies.* Thousand Oaks, Calif.: Pine Forge Press.

Morgan, R., L. (1990). *No wrinkles on the soul.* Nashville: Upper Room Books.

Neugarten, B., L. (1977). Personality and aging. In *Handbook of the psychology of aging,* ed. J. E. Birren and K. W. Schaie, 626–49. New York: Van Nostrand Reinhold.

Payne, B., and E. Brewer, eds. (1989). *Gerontology in theological education.* New York: Hawthorne Press.

Smith, J. M. (1993). Function and supportive roles of church and religion. In *Aging in black America,* ed. J. Jackson, L. Chatters and R. Taylor, 124–47. Beverly Hills, Calif.: Sage.

Taylor, R. J. (1993). Religion and religious observances. In *Aging in black America,* ed. J. Jackson, L. Chatters, and R. Taylor, 101–23. Beverly Hills, Calif.: Sage.

Tobin, S. S. (1985). Older Americans as a resource. In *Aging: Issues and policies for the 80's,* ed. T. Tedrick, 30–50. New York: Praeger.

Tobin, S. S., J. W. Ellor, and S. Anderson-Ray. (1986). *Enabling the elderly.* Albany: State University of New York Press.

Tirrito, T., and G. L. Euster. (1993). Gerontological education for religious leaders: Are they ready for the graying of the church? Paper presented at the Association for Gerontology in Higher Education conference, Louisville, Ky.

Turner, F., ed. (1992). *Mental health and the elderly.* New York: Free Press.

U.S. Bureau of the Census. (1990). *Statistical abstract of the United States,* 111th ed. Washington, D.C.: U.S. Government Printing Office.

Chapter 7

CULTURAL COMPETENCY
The Impact of Ethnicity and the Need for Services

A disproportionately large number of older Americans are members of an ethnic minority, and, as this population increases, physicians, lawyers, health care workers, and other professionals and organizations within the community must deal with increasing numbers of minority elderly patients and clients. Efforts of caregivers and service providers are frequently frustrated by having no shared language with the person they are attempting to serve as well as by cultural differences in background, economic status, and style of communication. Changes in curricula for professionals as well as the institution of in-service educational programs are needed if minority older adults are to receive optimal, effective services.

Although the focus of this book is on the independent practice arena, this chapter emphasizes the impact of the agency manager or health care administrator on shaping policy in this area of cultural competency. This is in recognition of the centrality of agency-based community services in the lives of the minority population. Furthermore, it is recognition of the influence of institutional policies on shaping the practices of independent service providers. The policies of professional educational and planning groups set the tone for practice on the level of the independent service provider. Professional educational and membership societies must be engaged in promoting cultural competency as well as in institutionalizing standards of interprofessional collaboration.

The turn-of-the-century view of America as a "melting pot," in which new immigrants attempted to jettison their old languages and cultures as quickly as possible in favor of a new language and new ways, has given way to recognition of ethnic and cultural diversity but with a common cause. People today tend more to be proud of their ethnic diversity and cultural heritage, recognizing that equality need not equal uniformity. This emphasis on cultural identity as an essential part of each individual has required increasing accommodation on the part of the caregiver or service provider, who, more often than not, is a member of a different ethnic group, has a different cultural orientation, and comes from a different educational and economic background from that of the person he or she is attempting to serve. This interesting phenomenon is fast moving from the intriguing to the urgent in the health care and legal sectors of our society, among others, as providers of services essential to the elderly face a rapidly growing older population, in which minorities are overrepresented. The fact that many of these minority old persons are also poor and in need of services from public agencies means that the caseloads of those serving such individuals are disproportionately filled with minority elderly. That these people have a right to optimal service is clear; that the care providers are committed to delivering the best services they can is, it is hoped, also clear. The question becomes: How can this challenge be met? In a climate of worldwide economic difficulty, in which obtaining maximum performance from existing resources is essential, what can be done to improve service to the minority elderly within the boundaries of the existing structure, so as to make these services "culturally competent"?

The areas in which culturally competent service is essential encompass all those services that involve the minority elderly, among them social services, including preventive and primary medical care; and long-term and hospice care; rehabilitation care and legal services.

The service environment or formal support system is composed of professionals and bureaucracies serving older adults and their families. One segment of this service environment consists of the human service organizations. The social worker's area of expertise represents but one aspect of the client's total situation, the psychosocial component. Another segment of the service environment of the older client is the professional community of physicians, dentists, allied health professionals, and lawyers in private practice. Wherever issues of autonomy, competence, and informed consent are raised, attention to cross-cultural perspectives is imperative. Medical assessments and legal directives about living wills or durable power of attorney, for instance, need to incorporate the views of the minority elderly about life, death, and spirituality, because these factors may influence the decisions that must be made. Gender roles, kin networks, and the diversity of people within specific cultural groups must also be acknowledged when addressing issues of autonomy and competence. In order to address the needs of the minority elderly, social workers and other professionals must develop culturally competent service delivery—that is, they must be familiar with the subcultures of the people to be served; with their social conditions, needs, and problems in a cross-cultural environment; and with the varied modes of intervention applicable to minority older adults.

THE PROBLEMS IN SERVICE DELIVERY
TO MINORITY OLDER ADULTS

The Client May Not Know What Services Are Available

The minority client and the client's family may be unaware of his or her entitlements. Many clients represent minority groups, which have historically been excluded from public services and are unaccustomed to accessing health, legal, or social services, if they or their families even know such services exist. Such lack of awareness may be foreign to the service provider, who daily deals with the provision or enabling of such services, and an explanation of the services and entitlements available to the client may receive short shrift. In dealing with the minority elderly it is best never to assume that the client is aware of what services are available but, rather, to take the time, in every case, to explain benefits and services thoroughly to both the client and his or her family.

Other minority older adults may be aware of available services but may be culturally indoctrinated to believe that accessing public services is somehow demeaning, even when such services are sorely needed. They may thus not seek aid or may shun it when it is offered, because of the way they perceive it. It therefore falls upon the caretaker or service provider to interact with the client in such a way that the client feels reassured in availing him- or herself of the services needed.

These points seem obvious and would, indeed, be so to the sensitive, conscientious caretaker or service provider. Yet, in dealing with minority elderly, the multiple problems present in the management of elderly clients generally are further complicated by a number of factors. The provider and the client frequently share no common language; the client's degree of poverty and lack of education may be totally outside the frame of experience of the service provider, and, therefore, the client's problems or their significance to his or her life may not be adequately viewed or understood; the client may have such inadequate access to supportive resources that it is virtually impossible for him or her to take advantage of the services available. Although sensitivity to the cultural and ethnic background and values of the client is certainly essential in all cases, it becomes an ethical imperative when caring for minority elderly, for which cultural competence may represent the largest, most important factor in effective delivery of services to the client.

The Client May Not Be Able to Access His or Her Entitlements

Language difficulties. Very often the client or patient and the care or service provider share no common language and are completely unable to communicate verbally without the services of a third person, an interpreter, who can translate the interaction. Communicating with a client through a third party introduces a variety of potential problems into the relationship. First, the provider may tend to interact, or seem to interact, more with the interpreter than with the client or patient, leaving the latter with the feeling that he or she is being excluded from the exchange. This feeling of detachment, or remoteness, from the caregiver can sabotage the bond of trust which must be established between the service provider and client if an optimal working relationship is to be achieved. Second, even if the service provider has acquired some background, perhaps in high school or college, in the client's native tongue, the vocabulary and word usage of the client may make communication virtually impossible. The client may speak a regional dialect or nonstandard version of his or her own language which is unintelligible to the care provider, who has likely learned the formal language in school, and thus the client may feel self-conscious and ill at ease, even ashamed, dealing with the provider. Additionally, the culture of the client may mandate an entirely different "style" of verbal communication from that with which the provider is familiar, so that important messages may not be communicated or may be communicated in such a manner that the other person fails to understand the importance of what is being said.

Transportation and financial difficulties. The middle-class professional who is attempting to deliver services to a minority elderly client may, because of lack of exposure, fail to comprehend the nature or seriousness of the problems encountered by that client in such very basic areas as arriving at a given site punctually for an appointment. If the client must depend on relatives, neighbors, or friends for transportation, he or she often must conform to their schedules and may be extremely restricted in setting appointments. Additionally, the punctuality with which the client is able to arrive at an appointment may then depend on a variety of factors: the importance of punctuality, as a concept, to the person providing transportation (and the need for punctuality is often quite different across various cultures), the importance of the client's appointment in the eyes of the transportation provider, how comfortable the client is with expressing his or her need to be punctual to the person providing transportation, and so on. Should the caregiver insist that the client be punctual in a situation in which the client has no control over that punctuality or in which the client's insistence, to the transportation provider, on punctuality may compromise a relationship important to the client, the entire relationship between care provider and client may be jeopardized. The client may give up on obtaining needed services, feeling the stakes are simply too high. Should a provider suggest to the client that he or she "take a cab," the client may be too embarrassed to admit that he or she has insufficient funds to do so.

Value conflicts within the client's family. Frequently, an older minority client, and his or her opinions and decisions, were once highly revered within the family but now are disregarded because the older adult has become dependent upon his or her children or grandchildren. It is not uncommon for the younger generations, more assimilated into the dominant culture and eager to conform to its manners and mores, to regard their elders as old-fashioned and out of touch. When communication with the client must be "filtered" through such a young person, it can be extremely difficult for the caregiver to determine what the wishes of the client are vis-à-vis the opinions and desires of the younger family member. Such an interpreter, whether consciously or inadvertently, may alter the translation and/or interpretation of the information being transmitted. It may be that the young person finds the wishes of the older person inconvenient to his or her own lifestyle, or it could be that, in a wish to conform to the expectations of the caregiver, the younger family member is embarrassed by what the older person has actually expressed.

Sex-based differences between the client and the interpreter can also impede the accurate transmission of what the client is attempting to express. If the interpreter is not of the same sex as the patient or client, either the minority elderly person may be unwilling to express him- or herself frankly and openly, or the interpreter may be reluctant to transmit the information fully, through embarrassment or self-consciousness.

The Caregiving System May Label the Minority Older Adult as "Difficult"

Fineman, in 1991, investigated noncompliance in a cross-cultural, multiservice senior center, as it was defined by staff members, including physicians, nurses, and social workers. He found noncompliance to be socially constructed and subjectively defined and interpreted. Caretakers defined behavior as compliant when it followed their expectations; when behavior deviated from those expectations, it was defined as noncompliant. The staff, in addition to expecting health-appropriate behavior, assumed clients would be "honest, punctual, cooperative, reasonable, responsible, self-aware, self-interested, polite, open-minded and supportive of staff's efforts."

In nursing literature considerable confirmation can be found for the premise that the minority elderly are frequently labeled "difficult," or "problem," patients (Chandy et al. 1987; Leininger 1984; Slocum 1989). Difficult patients are synonymous with noncompliant patients and are, therefore, labeled "complaining," "demanding," and "abusive" (English and Morse 1988). Kim (1983) described how a Chinese patient suffering from symptomatic hypocalcemia who had refused treatment with calcium supplements and dietary milk products—a reasonable response, given his distaste for milk and the high rate of lactose intolerance among Asians—was labeled "stubborn" and "responsible for prolonging his illness."

Cross-cultural expectations, if they are not understood, can promote frustration, anger, and emotional withdrawal and distancing in the caregiving relationship, destroying the bond of trust so essential to effective delivery of services to the minority elderly.

THE MEANING OF CULTURAL COMPETENCE
TO THE SERVICE PROVIDER

Understanding Cultural Diversity in Communication

If the caregiver or service provider is to work effectively with the minority elderly, he or she must understand the client's culturally defined behavior, both within his or her informal support network and during the professional intervention. To do this the service provider must be aware of the general cultural background of the client's ethnic group and be sensitive to the differences that exist between the values of the client and the values of the caregiver. This sensitivity and awareness must exist in both a general sense and within the particular interaction taking place. Although the progression for development of this sensitivity is not ordered in any formal way, logic would dictate that general concepts first be addressed, so as to provide a frame of reference for the more individualized aspects of cultural diversity.

We have mentioned the difficulties that can arise between the caregiver and the patient or client, owing to the two individuals sharing no common language. Effective communication, however, consists of much more than mere comprehension of the words being said, and the importance of these other factors—for example, the style of communication and the cultural appropriateness of communication—although always important, loom extremely large in interactions with the minority elderly client, in which what is not expressed in words may be more important than the verbal message. Generally, both parties to such a cross-cultural interaction, in their eagerness to understand the other, are particularly alert to the subtleties of interaction which may pass unnoticed in exchanges between people who have no such barriers to communication.

Overaccommodation may convey a lack of respect for the competence and status of the client and may make the professional appear patronizing. On the other hand, insufficient accommodation may leave the client with the impression that the professional is insufficiently interested in his or her well-being. The difficulty of maintaining a proper balance between nurturance and respect may cause either the professional or the client, or both, to cut short or avoid opportunities for communication, seriously damaging the ability of the caregiver to provide and the client to accept much-needed services (Wiemann et al. 1986).

The problems of older adults are emotionally charged. Major issues, such as dependence versus autonomy, declining physical health, acceptance of old age, dying and death, among others, confront an elderly client at every turn, and understanding the client's culturally oriented view of these issues is vital to a care provider who wishes to provide optimal services to the minority elderly patient or client. Often the client's cultural viewpoint about care may be at odds with what the provider has been schooled to believe is essential. For instance, a provider may urge a client to discuss, frankly and openly, the emotionally laden issues with which the client is obviously grappling. Such personal disclosure or any display of strong emotions with a stranger, however, is perceived as inappropriate behavior among many elderly from diverse ethnic backgrounds. A caregiver, eager to underscore the client's autonomy and self-esteem, may urge an elderly client to take responsibility for his health and health care, social welfare, or legal care, yet this behavior may be inconsistent with cultural and family traditions and mores. If the professional, confident that such acceptance of personal responsibility on the part of his client can be only beneficial, discounts these traditions, the result may be frustration and withdrawal on the part of the client. This behavior, in turn, may be regarded by a middle-class professional, for example, as unwillingness or reluctance, on the part of the client, to cooperate in what the caregiver regards as a necessary and helpful enterprise.

It may be difficult for the relatively youthful middle-class professional, raised in a society that is highly mobile and consists chiefly of nuclear families, to understand the role played by the extended family and close associates of the elderly minority client. In a time and a society when no governmental or private organizations existed to serve the elderly, and in which one's survival in old age depended solely upon one's extended family or other members of a close-knit community group, adaptation to the patterns of thought, belief, and action by these local cultural groups assumed a pivotal role. Quite literally, persons were enabled to survive, or they perished, according to their degree of conformity to and assimilation by the group. A minority elderly client who, in earlier years, found his or her security and safety in conformity to the mores of the societal group and who now feels an increasing need, in the vulnerability of his or her old age, for such support, may feel extremely threatened by the urging of the care provider toward greater autonomy.

The multiple choices offered by the professional may be perceived as bewildering, confusing, and even threatening rather than as opportunities that are potentially liberating. At precisely the time in life when the client most needs to feel secure and safe, the professional seems to be encouraging the individual to abandon those beliefs and customs that have served the client well for all of his or her life. Nonetheless, the professional must proceed with what he or she believes to be in the best interests of the patient or client, always striving for an appropriate balance between respect and nurturance. Overaccommodation can be perceived as patronizing and as demonstrating a lack of respect for the competence and status of the elderly client; insufficient accommodation may be seen by the client as showing a lack of interest and concern for his or her well-being. The difficulty of maintaining the proper balance between respect and nurturance may lead to overly brief professional exchanges with an elder or talking with a relative about the older person (when the older person is present) instead of speaking with the person directly, a practice certain to make the elderly individual feel discounted.

Understanding the Cultural Mores of the Client or Patient

If the previous comments make the demands for culturally competent service delivery to the minority elderly client seem overwhelming, it should be stated that the rewards are as great as the challenge. Over and above the satisfaction of having helped an elderly person toward greater dignity and an improved standard of living at a time of life when he or she may be beset with difficulties and problems, there is the chance to come to know another human being who has a very different background and belief system and the opportunity for both the caregiver and care recipient to grow, change, and enrich their own lives. The bond of shared humanity—of trust, mutual respect, and concern—which can arise in such an interaction is, in itself, sufficient reward for the efforts entailed, quite apart from the fact that it is the job of the service worker to provide services and of the caregiver to give care, both in the most effective manner possible.

The primary issue is, quite clearly, one of establishing trust, yet this is a goal for which it is difficult to compose guidelines. A "checklist of communication skills" for professionals working with the elderly in cross-cultural environments, which includes the following features, provides a useful evaluation tool for all professionals in both health care and social services (Harris and Moran 1979).

Respect and empathy. A professional schooled to expect respect from clients or patients must develop the ability to express respect for the client if effective and meaningful relations between caregiver and recipient are to develop. Clients and caregivers develop a rapport when they appear to understand things from similar viewpoints and are not battling for value supremacy.

Tolerating ambiguity. Inherent in cross-cultural interactions are dynamics that must be acknowledged, adjusted to, and accepted. The social service or health care provider must learn to react appropriately to new, different, and/or unpredictable situations arising from attention to the client's values, which often reflect an ethnic group's responses to the accessibility or delivery of the health and social service systems. Cultural competence implies an understanding of cultural preferences in order for the professional to be able to support client self-determination.

Being nonjudgmental. The professional must develop the ability to withhold judgment and remain objective until he or she has enough information about an alternative model of care being proffered by the client, family, and/or cultural environment. Inherent in the development of this attitude is the recognition that there is seldom only *the* way being prescribed by the professional. Cultural competence functions with an acceptance of a client's cultural "location" and adapts service delivery to accommodate the context within which the client functions.

Perseverance. The culturally competent professional may not be successful in communicating with the aged minority client upon initial intake, but, with practice and persistence, the understanding portion of the communication task can be accomplished.

Understanding the role played by one's own expectations. Perhaps the first and most important step in becoming culturally competent lies in an examination, by the service provider or caregiver, of his or her own expectations and an understanding of the role these expectations play in any interactions between the provider and the elderly client. Unfulfilled expectations on the part of the service provider can, as previously discussed, lead to labeling the client as noncompliant and his or her behavior as inappropriate and unreasonable, when, in reality, the behavior demonstrated may be completely acceptable within the client's cultural background, a background with which the caregiver likely is unfamiliar. Is the patient consistently late for appointments? Does the client fail to notify the service provider if he or she is unable to keep an appointment? Has the patient not filled the prescription given to him or her or not taken medication consistently or as directed? A well-intentioned, yet culturally different, client, because of his or her particular cultural frame of reference, may not even

103

understand why a service provider finds any of the client's reactions abnormal. Labeling a patient as uncooperative or noncompliant as a result of the care provider's unfulfilled expectations can destroy the trust so necessary for effective interaction, leaving both parties frustrated and negating any possibility for a successful future relationship.

Social workers, long accustomed to the need for effective communication with a client if optimal service is to be provided, will find nothing surprising in the demand for cultural competence as a way of enhancing the effectiveness of an interaction. Yet the need for cultural competence reaches much farther in the community, into many other professions and occupations. The needs of the culturally diverse are as complex and far-reaching as those of mainstream citizens, and, wherever services and/or care are to be delivered, cultural competence becomes essential, if the minority elderly person is to receive the services and/or care to which he or she is entitled.

Lawyers

Among the elderly seeking legal representation, certain themes recur, and certain problems emerge again and again. The minority elderly constitute a large portion of those elderly in need of legal services. The problems facing an elderly minority person seeking legal advice are twofold. First, many lawyers have not been well prepared for service to the elderly. Very often law school and private practice have not prepared attorneys for the intricacies of government benefit programs, issues about immigration and citizenship status, and the moral and legal issues involved in terminating life-support systems (Regan 1990). Second, barriers such as language, lack of finances, lack of trust, and fear of self-disclosure compound the legal problems of the minority elderly.

A new legal specialty has been developed, covering the spectrum of legal issues facing many older Americans, called "elder law." Attorneys who represent and advise elders are strongly encouraged to inform themselves about and to practice elder law, in order to provide optimal services to their clients. Elder law work requires a detailed knowledge of public benefit programs, including Medicaid, Social Security, Medicare, Supplemental Security Income (SSI), in-home support services, and housing for the elderly. Attorneys today encounter a growing demand from elderly clients of all income levels for advice on issues as varied as entitlement to Medicare benefits, estate planning, and the right to die. Regan (1992) views the dominant theme of elder practice as empowerment of the client through a knowledgeable and sensitive representation of his or her interests. Many in the "sandwich" generation (those who are raising their children and simultaneously caring for aged parents) are seeking advice for their

104

parents in making decisions prompted by retirement, program entitlements, and/ or nursing home placement. Income, housing, health care, entitlements, and estate planning are all issues that present difficult legal impasses for the elderly and their families.

The Rules of Professional Conduct honor the right to self-determination by encouraging the development of attorney-client relationships despite limitations on a client's capacity, thus limiting interference with a client's autonomy. "The lawyer's duty is to advocate the wishes of the client and the client is entitled to reasonable competence, preparation, and communication in the presentation" (*Nebraska State Bar Association v. Walsh* 1980). These issues are a given for all clients, but in light of minority elders' negative experiences in accessing the social welfare and health care systems, the problem of culturally competent, empathetic lawyers becomes even more urgent.

It is vital that the attorney remember *who the client is* and not allow children, spouses, or others to speak for the older person. It is equally important that the attorney's considerations about an elderly client's potential capacity not be tainted by stereotypes or the attorney's own attitudes about aging and motivation. "Examination of one's own attitudes about aging and motivations and interactions with older clients is an important first step in being able to work effectively with older persons" (Hommel 1986). Hommel recommends the following techniques in interviewing elderly persons: develop trust and confidence; beware of conflicts of interest and paternalism; sharpen listening skills; avoid dependence; actively involve the client and maintain contact; organize sessions and times carefully; know how to close an interview in the attorney-client relationship; and learn about community resources for older people.

Physicians

There is strong evidence that few doctors want to work with elderly patients and that this aversion to caring for the elderly will continue (Institute of Medicine 1987). Many researchers have found that doctors, medical students, residents, and other health care providers prefer to work with younger patient groups rather than caring for the elderly (Merrill and Laux 1987). With the elderly currently making up 13 percent of the U.S. population, and steadily increasing, this problem, already acute, is in danger of becoming catastrophic. In the medical profession, therefore, the movement toward cultural competence in dealing with the minority elderly must be preceded or accompanied by a reeducation process, if physicians are to be willing to treat the elderly at all. Medical schools and the medical community need to develop creative educational programs geared toward reversing ageist attitudes and promoting cul-

105

tural competence in future medical practitioners as well as raising the consciousness level among those physicians already in practice.

All too often a medical student experiences his or her first exposure to older persons in a hospital geriatric service or nursing home, where the student encounters only frail, chronically ill, acutely ill, or otherwise incapacitated elderly persons. Physicians are taught to be problem solvers; thus, it is easy to understand their aversion to dealing with the elderly if all they see, when they look at an elderly person, is an unsolvable problem—inexorable physical decline ending in death. If medical students were introduced to relatively well elderly people before they encounter those who are ill or incapacitated, through interaction with and personal service to older people living in the community near the medical school, students' views about the elderly would be more well-rounded. A program such as the "buddy system" (Langer 1993) would help in reversing negative attitudes by providing both the medical student and the elderly mentor with personal, intellectual, and social stimuli through students' visits and interactions.

The tendency, because of their training, of physicians to see a medical problem as a scientific dilemma requiring a scientific solution often prompts a medical professional to attempt to cure or treat a physical condition without regard for the patient's emotional or cultural needs. Cultural competence among physicians will, therefore, positively impact the care given the aged minority patient, by encouraging understanding of the patient's long-standing attitudes and beliefs about health, illness, and dying, beliefs that largely determine the patient's behavior and coping style. If ethnically diverse patients are to be treated effectively, physicians must respect the patient's cultural view of symptoms, etiology, diagnosis, health-seeking behavior, treatment, and medication and come to tolerate and practice a holistic approach to health and illness. Alternative healing methods that are valid for the patient—for example, indigenous healers, herbal remedies, acupuncture, spiritual healing, among others—must be accepted as important to the patient's state of health or healing and must be dealt with, by the physician, with an attitude of respect. The sensitive medical practitioner will appreciate the cultural relevance of the nonmedical model, understand its importance to the patient, and therefore to the patient's health, and accept that it can coexist with his or her practice of modern scientific medicine.

Dentists

Dental practitioners, like physicians, must come to see their patients, not just as medical problems requiring solutions but, rather, as whole human beings whose cultural beliefs and attitudes influence their health and their ways of seeking and obtaining health care. A dentist practicing culturally competent care of the minority elderly patient will take into account that such a patient may have been unable to afford preventive dental care in the past and may be visiting a dentist for the first time in his or her life. Many people fear dental procedures, even if they have had regular dental care since childhood. This commonplace fear can be greatly amplified in the minority elderly patient who experiences communication barriers, who has had little or no prior experience with a dentist, and who has a lack of trust toward authority figures or feels patronized or denigrated because of belonging to an ethnically diverse group. A dentist who takes the time to understand the cultural component of such a patient's anxieties and exercises sensitivity in addressing his or her fears can greatly impact the positive aspects of the patient's experience and influence whether this patient will seek and accept future dental care.

Other Service Providers

Although many of the major decisions concerning the welfare of the minority elderly take place through contacts with social workers, physicians, dentists, lawyers, and other advocates or caregivers specifically geared toward providing services to this group, the ethnically diverse elderly interact with many other individuals and agencies within the community. If the minority elderly are to be well served, the need for awareness and understanding of and sensitivity toward ethnic diversity must extend to all sectors of the community. Elderly minority persons interact with banks and stores, insurance companies and public utilities, notaries and newspapers—the same people we all must deal with on a daily basis—but with the added difficulties presented by ethnic difference. Often, the resulting impaired communication causes both parties to the would-be transaction to become frustrated and annoyed, causing further reinforcement of existing prejudices and stereotypes.

Where to Begin

Just as prejudices and stereotypical thinking can be reinforced by ineffective interaction between two ethnically diverse individuals, so cultural competence can be a self-fulfilling endeavor that reinforces those elements common to the two sides of the interaction, substituting understanding and respect for old biases. The question, then, is not "Do we begin?" or "Is it worthwhile to begin?" but, rather, "Where do we begin?"

Cultural competence must be viewed not as a project with a beginning and an end but, instead, as a developmental process that is never complete and one that extends into all areas, at every level, of care and service provision. "A culturally competent system of care acknowledges and incorporates at all levels the importance of culture, the expansion of cultural knowledge, concern from the dynamics that result from cultural differences, and the adaptation of services to meet culturally unique needs" (Focal Point 1988).

Management must lead the way through attitude and action. When a social work or allied health care agency administrator, law firm partner, or director of a hospital residency program projects a sense of priority and understanding of the need for a culturally competent system of service provision, he or she sets the tone for the evolution of a culturally competent environment. If cultural competence is not a priority of the nursing supervisor of a community hospital or the curriculum committee of a medical school, then it will not be a priority with those actually delivering the care or teaching the curriculum. "Selling" a program of cultural competence must, therefore, begin "at the top."

Barriers to effective interaction with those who are ethnically different may evolve from the life experience of managers and professionals themselves. The problems one has in communicating with people different from ourselves may reflect previous experiences, or a lack thereof, in dealing with diversity. To the many agencies and professional practices predominantly managed by white males, older clients of diverse cultural backgrounds may seem completely alien. Education in the particulars of the culture in question, as well as in sensitivity to the types of issues of vital importance to older adults, regardless of cultural background, can go far toward explaining behavior and providing insight into why previous attempts at interaction may have failed or proved to be less than ideal.

Many professionals, particularly physicians and lawyers, have been schooled to treat all patients or clients precisely the same way, regardless of their backgrounds. Presenting the idea of "equitable" rather than "identical" treatment of patients and clients may therefore meet with initial resistance; however, it is physicians and lawyers, caught as they are in the perception of their patient's and client's problems as abstractions, who will benefit most from providing culturally competent care.

It cannot be denied that sometimes ethnic differences can and do present problems to the organizations and service environments attempting to provide for their needs. Yet understanding the cultural heritage and background, beliefs, and behaviors of the ethnically diverse can also strengthen those organizations whose goals include a value orientation toward diversity within equality.

It is not enough for management simply to pay lip service to "politically correct" racial, gender, and age policies within organizations focused on attaining cultural competence, nor is it enough for management to be convinced that achieving cultural competence is a desirable goal. Certainly, the latter is necessary, but it is not sufficient to bring about the changes that must be made for an organization to deliver culturally competent service. It is generally not, after all, the manager who delivers the service and who interacts with the patient or client.

Communicating Management's Intent

First, the rank and file of the organization—those foot soldiers who actually deal, on a day-to-day basis, with the elderly minority—must be informed of management's belief in the importance of cultural competence and of management's intent to institute practices that will change the organization in a way that is geared toward cultural competence. It does little good to ask people to undertake learning and performing a new task if they are not first convinced that the task occupies a top priority and its pursuit will be encouraged and monitored in a way that prompts the actual service providers to have an interest in carrying out the new policy.

Analysis of the Task

Ethnic diversity is not always understood and/or accepted by those who make policy and provide care for the elderly. It is not enough to focus on the professional interpretation of what kind of service is to be provided and how it is to be delivered. Cultural factors must also be taken into account in studying the aging process and in determining the perception of the minority elderly, in terms of what they believe their need for service to be and the manner in which its delivery is acceptable to them. Input from leaders of the ethnic community can be invaluable here; seeking such input can also impact favorably upon the members of the extended ethnic community at large, giving them the satisfaction of knowing that their interests and concerns matter and are being considered. The point, after all, is to improve conditions for the minority elderly person, as he or she perceives the quality of life, not just to satisfy the values of service providers. The changes needed to accommodate a particular ethnic group may be as major as the complete restructuring of how an organization provides services or as minor as having a same-sex or same-minority representative available to counsel and assist the minority elderly. Whatever the adjustments or changes that must be undertaken, professionals must find their source and their mode of application in careful, sensitive consultation with members of the ethnic group in question, with additional input from the particular subgroup—in this case, the elderly—which is to be served.

Training for Managers

Having informed service personnel of the intended change in policy and interaction, managers must address the myths, stereotypes, and real cultural differences among minority elderly clients and their service providers. Managers are advised to learn how different influences affect the perceptions and frameworks of reality for both minority personnel and clients. Once these issues are identified, a manager can proceed to investigate organizational barriers that impede full client access to services. Managers must, then, be empowered to develop programs and delivery systems commensurate with client needs and must be held accountable for the effectiveness of these programs and systems.

A great deal of synergy takes place when managers acknowledge cultural diversity and help both personnel and clients to bridge gaps. Agencies can create multicultural health and social service resources by providing a learning area equipped with books, videos, and audiocassettes by experts in the field of health, social services, ethnic culture, and social gerontology. In-service training sessions can be instituted, in which formal lectures or the simple sharing of experiences can educate others and help them avoid cultural pitfalls.

Upward Mobility of Minority Managers

Because of the cultural identification they can bring to interactions with culturally diverse patients or clients, minority managers can be invaluable in the interface between the caregiving, service-providing establishment and the ethnically diverse. The potential contribution of minority managers must be recognized by the relevant organizations and encouraged through mentoring, formal training, executive appointment, and other programs. It is essential in the encouragement and promotion of minority managers that respect for the culturally diverse be emphasized and underscored. Particularly in dealing with minority elderly, identification of a minority manager may be less with the elderly individual than with the nonminority, mainstream establishment, to the detriment of any interactions between manager and client. Sensitivity to the dilemma of the minority manager in such a situation is essential; if the minority manager is uncomfortable in his or her role, beneficial interactions are less likely. It is the task of management to reassure a minority manager of the importance of his or her task to the organization as a whole and to encourage and reward success by this manager.

RECOGNITION OF BIAS EXISTING
AMONG SERVICE PROVIDERS

Although organizational change directed at cultural competence is possible and desirable and professional vision must be as broad as the client's environment, the limitations of service personnel's effectiveness must also be understood.

The irrationality characterizing our long-term system is deeply rooted in the values and beliefs of our society. American society's ambivalence in regard to institutional responses to human need illustrates the desire to provide adequate services and care while resenting the "freeloaders" who depend on public services. The implicit rationale of many publicly funded programs is social control and since minority elderly are often also our nation's poor, the implicit organizational mandate of social control is usually viewed in relation to this "disruptive" segment of the population. (Silverstone 1983, 230)

To the extent that the service provider is able to understand the patient or client as a whole individual, part and parcel of his cultural heritage and environment, this attitude may be ameliorated. Yet service providers are "whole people" too, and it is hardly appropriate (nor is it effective) for management to attempt to enforce, through dogmatic or dictatorial means, a program aimed at promoting greater sensitivity toward, and awareness of, other people only. It is therefore imperative that management be sensitive to the initial attitudes of personnel, by offering encouragement and empathy; it is hoped that such an attitude, coupled with patience and support, will lead to further understanding on the part of all those involved and the beginning of more empathetic, and thus more effective, interactions.

Those who value the concept of cultural competence must recognize that, no matter which measure is taken, leadership by top management is imperative. The cascade of attitudinal and behavioral change must begin at the top. Management must be convinced of the need for culturally competent service delivery and must actively pursue cultural competence as an organizational priority through programs designed to encourage constructive communication about differences both within the organization and within our ethnically diverse society. Effective measures must be instituted within the organization to support, encourage, guide, and reward effective intercultural interactions as a priority. Managers need to remind themselves and their staffs continuously that the difficult, sometimes threatening issues raised by cultural competence constitute no excuse for avoiding change; they must then gently, but persistently, pursue an unswerving plan of action directed toward greater cultural understanding and sensitivity in all interactions with the minority elderly.

Ethically responsible professionals must recognize that, even working within the confines of sometimes stifling organizational constraints, they have a responsibility to interact with minority elderly clients in a culturally competent manner, if they are to fulfill their ethical responsibilities to such clients. Often, the powerlessness and vulnerability of the minority elderly consumer are a function not only of his or her personal depletion but also of the status he or she is accorded within a given organizational structure. Minority elders are often helpless to influence the agencies and services upon which they are so dependent. Inflexible rules and policies may affect the way in which services are provided, restricting the freedom of clients and workers to individualize care plans. When agencies are organized so that feedback mechanisms are built into the structure, an ongoing process exists to accommodate changing population needs and to address problematic situations. If management is not 100 percent dedicated to the concept of cultural competence and to the reward of culturally competent employees, a care provider's reinforcement must come from the enriched interactions he or she will enjoy with the culturally diverse population, through his or her own efforts. Fortunately, as we have stated, culturally competent interactions bring with them their own reward in the personal enrichment gained by both parties.

Medical technology has responded to the needs of the aged population. Now social advocacy on behalf of the minority elderly must take up the task, if the last years of life are to have quality and dignity for them. Work with the aged has not been a popular pursuit for social workers and other professionals, and the problems inherent in interacting with the minority elderly compound this already difficult issue. In order to deliver optimal services to the minority elderly, professionals need to "climb inside the client's skin to understand empathically his [or her] feelings of psychological need and to form a relationship with him [or her]" (Wasser 1966). The minority elderly client has a right to have his or her sociocultural background understood and to have services provided within a framework that is meaningful to him or her.

To this end it is the responsibility of service organizations to examine, at a management level, how well their services and personnel provide for the minority elderly in a culturally relevant manner; to construct and initiate programs designed to promote culturally competent service delivery to the culturally diverse; and to reinforce the continued sensitivity among personnel to ethnic minority clients through regular review of practices, policies, and service delivery.

It is equally the responsibility of ethical individual service providers to maintain cultural competence and sensitivity in all their interactions with elderly minority clients and to remain mindful that, by addressing the elderly minority client's cultural needs, one is acknowledging that person's identity and right to self-determination. The challenge is to be scrupulously aware of the rights of the minority elderly and to humanize the resources and organizations that have been created to protect and service this community. Through education, training, and open communication a partnership between agencies and the minority elderly can be established.

REFERENCES

Chandy, J., T. L. Schwenk, L. D. Roi, and M. Cohen. (1987). Medical care and demographic characteristics of "difficult" patients. *Journal of Family Practice* 24, no. 6: 607–10.

English, J., and J. M. Morse. (1988). The "difficult" elderly patient: Adjustment or maladjustment? *International Journal of Nursing Studies* 25, no. 1: 23–39.

Fineman, N. (1991). The social construction of noncompliance: Implications for cross-cultural geriatric practice. *Journal of Cross-Cultural Gerontology* 6:219–27.

Focal Point. (1988). Vol. 3, no. 1 (Fall).

Harris, P. R., and R. T. Moran. (1979). *Managing cultural differences.* Houston: Gulf Publishing.

Hommel, M. (1986). Advising the elderly client. Committee on Continuing Legal Education of the State Bar of South Dakota.

Institute of Medicine. (1987). Academic geriatrics for the year 2000. *New England Journal of Medicine* 316:1425–28.

Kim, S. S. (1983). Ethnic elders and American health care: A physician's perspective. *Western Journal of Medicine* 139, no. 6: 81–87.

Langer, N. (1993). Medical practitioner geriatric training through a buddy system. AGHE presentation. Louisville, Ky.

Leininger, M. (1984). Transcultural nursing: An overview. *Nursing Outlook* 32, no. 2: 72–73.

Merrill, J. M., and L. Laux. (1987). Why medical students shun the elderly. *Clinical Research* 34:317A.

Nebraska State Bar Association v. Walsh. 1980. 294 N.W. 2d 873.

Travis, J. (1993). New piece in Alzheimer's puzzle. *Science* 261:828–29.

Regan, J. J. (1992). *Tax, estate, and financial planning for the elderly.* New York: Matthew Bender.

———. (1990). *The aged client and the law.* New York: Columbia University Press.

Silverstone, B. (1983). *Social work practice with the frail elderly and their families.* Springfield, Ill.: Charles C. Thomas.

Slocum, H. (1980). "Not him again": Thoughts on coping with irritating elderly patients. *Geriatrics* 44, no. 10: 75–84.

Wasser, E. (1966). *Creative approaches in casework with the aging.* New York: Family Service Association of America.

Wiemann, J. M., N. Coupland, H. Giles, K. Henwood, P. Rowlands, and W. Coupland. (1986). Beliefs about talk: Intergenerational perspectives. Paper presented at the annual meeting of the Speech Communication Association, Boston, November.

Chapter 8

SOCIAL FUNCTIONING
Assessment and Impact on the Need for Services

In old age, as in childhood, life presents the individual with the need to adapt to a series of changes. For children the changes represent an opportunity for exploration and independence, greater physical strength, growing skills, and the expansion of once limited horizons. For older adults the changes commonly bring just the opposite: fewer opportunities, lessened independence, a shrinking of the individual's feeling of competence and self-esteem, and physical frailty. Children, it is hoped, have the ongoing support of parents, other relatives, and peers—people who love and care for them, who have experienced the self-same changes they are undergoing, and who can offer assurance in times of their self-doubt or difficulty. Elderly persons all too often may have outlived spouses, family members, and friends and have no one who cares or can empathize, through shared experience, with the pain, fear, and loss they are experiencing. Yet every human being, whatever the stage of life, has a need for love, support, empathy, and reassurance. Often for the elderly these needs must be filled by formal social services, yet many of the most needy and vulnerable elderly do not access this vital lifeline. Who are these vulnerable elderly? Why are they vulnerable? Why are they not "connected" to the system of services available, and how can this linkage be enabled and made effective?

COMPONENTS OF SOCIAL FUNCTIONING

Needs, Resources, Person, Environment

Enhancing social functioning involves addressing common human needs that must be adequately met if individuals are to achieve a reasonable degree of

115

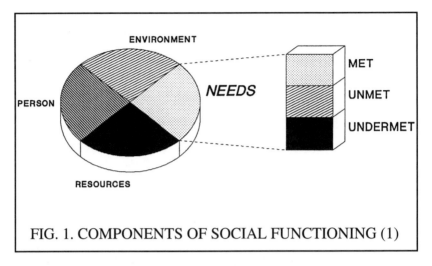

FIG. 1. COMPONENTS OF SOCIAL FUNCTIONING (1)

fulfillment and function as productive and contributing members of society. Human needs will necessarily include self-esteem and self-confidence; feelings of being needed and valued by others as well as a sense of belonging; personal fulfillment as a result of accomplishment; and basic physical needs of food, clothing, housing, health care, and safety (Hepworth 1993) (see fig. 1). In order to meet human needs, essential resources and opportunities must be available. The unmet and undermet needs constitute the incongruities of social institutions and systems in adequately matching needs to resources. The aim of social work, according to Rosenfeld, "is to match resources with needs to increase the 'goodness of fit' between them" (Rosenfeld 1983). Resources, however, even when they are available, are often underused by elderly clients, who are unaware of available services, cannot utilize them when they are available, or refuse to access services (see fig. 2).

When environments are rich in resources required for prevention (e.g., the timely provision of services to at-risk elderly before the onset of debilitating dysfunction), restoration (e.g., the physical, mental, and/or social rehabilitation of clients), and remediation (e.g., elimination or amelioration of an existing problem), the elderly can, within limits, continue to function. When environments lack vital resources, the physical, social, and emotional development of the individual is compromised, and social functioning may be adversely affected. Gaps in the environmental resources, deficiencies in individuals who need or utilize these resources, or dysfunctional transactions between individu-

116

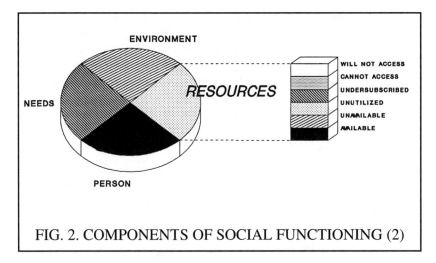

FIG. 2. COMPONENTS OF SOCIAL FUNCTIONING (2)

als and environmental systems block the fulfillment of human needs and lead to impaired functioning (Hepworth 1993) (see figs. 3 and 4). Frailty signals a life transition that "requires new responses from the environment" (Germain 1979). These responses are closely related to the multiple depletions suffered by the frail and their need for different and greater support from their environments. Professional community practice involves assisting vulnerable elderly to find ways to meet their needs by linking them with resources and/or providing coping mechanisms to deal with environmental factors.

When considering the social aspects of aging, one must focus on how older people function within a particular social structure and how they are affected by the society in which they live. Vital concerns are (1) the manner in which increased age affects social roles and status, (2) patterns of interpersonal relationship, and (3) patterns of interaction between the elderly and social institutions.

In old age social roles are frequently altered dramatically or are lost. This alteration in roles, whether through loss produced by retirement, change in specific family role, or loss of social position, very often impacts the elderly person adversely. Role and status are inseparable; therefore, role change or loss always produces status change or loss. Because social roles are basic to self-identity (Who am I?) and status (What am I worth? How am I valued?), the role/status changes that occur in later life pose a serious threat to an elderly person's psychological well-being, which, in turn, impacts his or her physical and further social well-being. Consider the following:

—A childless, widowed man (he had a son once, but his son was killed in Korea; he will proudly show you the medals), working as an office machines repairman for a large corporate office, is forced by the firm, finally, to retire. On the following Monday, however, he appears at his usual station at his usual time. He is willing to perform his accustomed tasks for no salary rather than sit alone, day after day, in a small inner-city apartment, with only his television for company. Gently, his supervisor, a man less than half his age, explains that he cannot come to his old job anymore. The old man cries.

—A young woman waits at a bus stop in front of the opera house in a large West Coast city, her arms laden with opera scores. A bent old woman approaches. "You're a singer, I see. You'll understand! I used to be the wig master there," she says, pointing. "I worked with all the great opera stars in my day. I was so busy," she smiles, "that I never had time to get married!" The young woman draws her out. The bus arrives, and, as the young woman makes her good-byes and turns away, the old woman says: "Thank you for listening to me. I did something important once, but nobody cares anymore. Sometimes I go for days without saying a word to anybody. I'm just a bothersome old woman now, and nobody wants to hear anything I have to say."

—An old woman wakes in her lonely farmhouse. Once there were the children. "Mom, I need a dozen cupcakes for the class bake sale tomor-

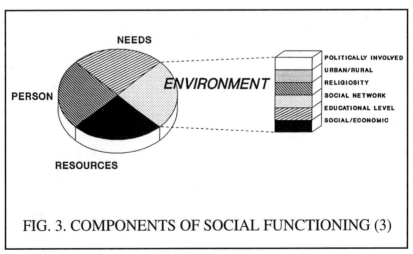

FIG. 3. COMPONENTS OF SOCIAL FUNCTIONING (3)

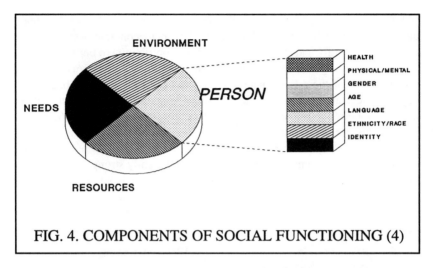

FIG. 4. COMPONENTS OF SOCIAL FUNCTIONING (4)

row." "Mom, can you help me with my history homework?" "Mom, I've just got to have a new prom dress. Can you sew it for me, if I help?" Then, there was her husband. "Nobody makes pot roast like you, Mama! You're the greatest. Is my new shirt ironed?" Now the children are far away, and her husband is dead. Maybe she just won't get up today. What's the use? She'll just have a bowl of cold cereal if she gets too hungry.

Loneliness is a serious issue for many older adults. Vital support networks diminish, as families move and significant others—spouses, relatives, friends, and neighbors—die. Economic and social disadvantages that have plagued at-risk groups increase and take on greater significance with older age. It took a lot of energy, all their lives, for these people to cope with these problems, and now they no longer have the energy or psychological resources to do so. The impact of race, ethnicity, and gender can produce "double" or "triple" jeopardy through lifelong decreasing access to economic opportunities, which is aggravated by aging (Hendricks and Hendricks 1986).

For many people the period following retirement occupies an increasing segment of the life cycle, as medical advances extend life. Older people's needs will change over this significant span of their lives, but many are ill prepared or completely unprepared for the biological, psychological, and social adjustments that will have to be made during this period.

Cath, a geriatric psychiatrist, has proposed a meaningful construct for professional community providers of the elderly. He states that, as people grow old, they share a need for basic anchorages, which include (1) an intact body and body image, (2) an acceptable home, (3) a socioeconomic base, and (4) a meaningful identity and purpose in life. Cath's contribution to our understanding of the challenges of the transitions and crises of aging in terms of loss or threat of loss of these basic anchorages is clear. As the multiple biological, psychological, and social losses accrue, older people and those who care about them are required to find compensations to restore stability (Cath 1963).

To illustrate, let us picture an old-fashioned wagon wheel having four necessary spokes: P = person; E = environment; N = needs; and R = resources (fig. 5). Only if there are enough spokes that are sufficiently strong can the wheel continue to turn and to support the weight of the wagon. Note that, in panel A, one spoke is broken; the individual has no contact with the social services system, because he or she does not presently perceive the need for services or

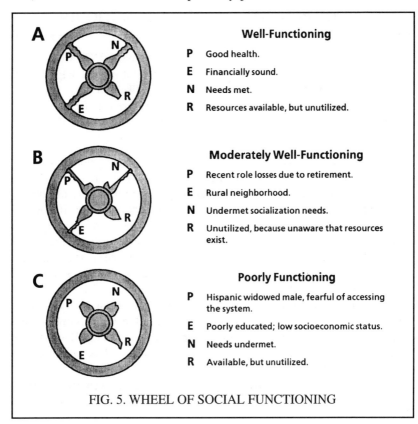

A

Well-Functioning

P   Good health.

E   Financially sound.

N   Needs met.

R   Resources available, but unutilized.

B

Moderately Well-Functioning

P   Recent role losses due to retirement.

E   Rural neighborhood.

N   Undermet socialization needs.

R   Unutilized, because unaware that resources exist.

C

Poorly Functioning

P   Hispanic widowed male, fearful of accessing the system.

E   Poorly educated; low socioeconomic status.

N   Needs undermet.

R   Available, but unutilized.

FIG. 5. WHEEL OF SOCIAL FUNCTIONING

realize there are any services available. Nonetheless, this wheel can continue to turn, so long as the remaining spokes remain intact. Yet, given the vicissitudes and degenerative changes of old age, the situation is unlikely to remain stable over time. Sooner or later other spokes will weaken or become damaged, and this wheel will no longer be able to support the wagon. In panel B only one spoke is broken—again, it is the contact to the social services system—but all of the other spokes are seriously compromised in strength. This wheel may be able to turn, but any serious "load" on the wagon will very likely cause one or more of the weakened spokes to break completely. This represents a person whose need is more urgent than the first, because, although the functional areas still exist, it is quite likely that a breakdown in functioning is not too far away. In panel C the wheel can no longer turn or support the wagon at all. This individual is in urgent need of immediate help. He or she simply has insufficient resources to function at even a minimal level. This man is one of the vulnerable elderly.

THE VULNERABILITY OF OLDER ADULTS
AND THEIR NEED FOR SOCIAL CONNECTIONS

When Family Is Unavailable or Geographically Distant

The oldest segment of the aged population, those most vulnerable to the need for care, has been growing at a more rapid rate than the total elderly population and will continue to do so during the next few decades. Historically, adult children, primarily daughters and daughters-in-law, have provided the vast majority of care services for the aged. Women's changing roles and lifestyles, specifically their rapidly increasing rate of entry into the labor force, will, in the future, make them less available as providers of certain concrete care services. Older people have not been abandoned by their children and other kin in the United States; closest to, and most involved in the daily life of the elderly, are the kin. U.S. society, however, has become highly mobile, and, as often as not, grown children live geographically quite distant from their parents. Overall, the trend toward greater residential separation between generations suggests that future cohorts of the elderly may have increasing proportions of distant children and other kin.

It is a frequent assumption in our society that most older men and women have children, grandchildren, and perhaps even great-grandchildren. Many couples, however, are electing not to have children, and this assumption may be farther afield than ever in the coming decades. Focus on the family should not obscure the fact that there are significant numbers of older people without children.

121

When the Family Has Rejected or Abandoned an Elderly Person

Much attention has been paid in recent years to the pain of children who have suffered abuse at the hands of their parents and subsequent alienation or to the distress of those who have adopted lifestyles that have caused their families to turn away from them. Although not a new phenomenon, the open admission that existing family may not be supportive reveals a group of older adults who have been, for the most part, previously ignored—those who have living family members but who receive no psychological or emotional support from them. These older adults are, in effect, without any family network at all. Aside from neighbors and friends, these individuals have only the formal support system to turn to.

Elderly Who Live in Rural Areas

Gerontological literature inconsistently reports differences between rural and urban families. Rural areas are depicted as pillars of traditional values, yet the results of research indicate that social services are needed particularly for health maintenance, household chores, personal care and grooming, and transportation (Goodfellow 1983). Studies have shown that, compared with urban older people, rural older adults have smaller incomes, are less mobile, experience poorer physical health, and have a more negative outlook on life (Scheidt 1984).

Elderly Who Have Historically Been Excluded

One might assume that utilization of social welfare services would be high among minority older adults because of their risk for poverty, poor health, cultural alienation, and other problems, yet this is not the case. Minority older adults do not receive a share of social welfare benefits in proportion to their needs (Cuellar and Weeks 1980). Studies have identified illiteracy, language problems, and economic and cultural roadblocks as hindering minority groups' access to services (Gelfand and Barresi 1987). Underutilization also occurs when services are interpreted to be insensitive to cultural differences (Markides and Mindel 1987).

Cultural barriers represent another reason for underutilization of social services. Lack of familiarity with services, fear of coercion or sanctions when accessing these services, and injury to personal pride at having to request services are important reasons for low utilization rates among minority older adults (Broderick 1988).

Uncompensated Losses

In old age the list of losses seems interminable and is constantly growing: loss of one's job-oriented role because of retirement; loss of one's family role through the death of a spouse; loss of social honor through societal disregard of the elderly; serious decline or loss of vital senses (e.g., hearing or sight); loss of health and vigor; and economic loss due to seriously diminished income once one's working days are past. In some cases an elderly individual has not previously perceived that a loss would be encountered, and so no preparations have been made. For example, a man who has worked all of his life at a job he merely tolerated may view prospective retirement with undiluted joy, as he looks forward to being freed of a longtime burden. He has little or no understanding that his former job had served to structure his time and to provide emotional stimulation as well as economic sustenance. The loss of his paycheck, loss of socialization with his coworkers, and the long, empty hours for which he has made no plans to fill represent an unanticipated and uncompensated loss.

Other losses arrive suddenly and perhaps totally without warning, such as the death of one's spouse. Like ripples in a formerly calm lake when a stone is thrown, the effects of such a loss widen until they encompass all areas of the individual's life. To an older woman the loss of her husband may precipitate economic disaster, if the couple has not made provisions for this event. Many poor older adults have been unable, during their productive years, to save sufficient funds to offset such a loss; further, some individuals are so frightened by considering death that they resolutely refuse to consider planning for such a loss. The day-to-day life of the surviving spouse may be disrupted in very basic, elemental ways. Who is to go to the grocery store or the pharmacy for needed supplies, if the surviving spouse is unable to drive? Who is to provide nourishing, well-balanced meals? In all marriages couples tend to adopt "roles" and to divide tasks more or less consistently; among the elderly such role-related division of tasks is often more rigid than for others. Thus, the surviving member of such a couple feels as if part of his or her very existence has been ripped away when a spouse dies.

Clearly, many losses cannot be anticipated, and the degree of one's ability to compensate for them is highly individualized. Those older persons who, for whatever reason, are unable to compensate for inevitable losses are considered the vulnerable elderly.

Personal Issues

The losses of old age are felt by all—rich or poor, healthy or sick, educated or uneducated—but the burden of compensating for or dealing with the inevitable problems varies considerably among individuals. Economic status is a powerful determinant of an elderly person's ability to cope; intelligence and education also play a considerable role, as does an individual's degree of physical and mental health. The vulnerable elderly are often shortchanged in a variety of areas, each of which impacts upon the others. A poor minority elderly person, for example, may not, in his or her lifetime, have had the funds or the education to seek needed medical care and thus arrives at old age with multiple medical problems that might have been staved off had circumstances been different. To a highly dependent individual who has never had to make important life decisions, losses encountered may seem insurmountable, whereas a person accustomed to taking charge in times of difficulty or crisis may be able to cope with problems far more easily.

PROBLEMS IN FORGING CONNECTIONS
WITH THE FORMAL SYSTEM

In the field of aging we may successfully argue the need for increased social and health services. Yet the greater problem may be our inability to deliver what we do have to those who need the services most. The at-risk elderly do not self-refer. If they receive help, it is because someone else obtained it for them. Traditional outreach efforts in aging programs have succeeded in providing access to the service system for older people who can seek help on their own or who have informal support networks working in their behalf. Such efforts, however, have been unsuccessful in reaching many of the vulnerable elderly.

The formal support system is an important part of the social environment; it consists of professionals in human service organizations who serve the elderly and their families. Although the focus of this book is on the independent practitioner, the authors recognize that community-based social services traditionally are delivered within a formal support system. These connections with the formal support system are elaborated in this chapter.

For many of the vulnerable elderly no effective family support system exists. When help is needed, this group has no one to turn to outside the formal support system. If connection with the formal support system is not achieved by or for these individuals, they will not receive help at all, often with disastrous results. And there are other, more subtle, if equally important, reasons for linking the vulnerable elderly with formal support systems.

One would think that, if a family support system does exist and this family support system exhibits high levels of intergenerational solidarity, high levels of psychological well-being in the elderly members of such a family would be present as well. Indeed, much of the literature on the subject suggests such a relationship. In 1985, however, Markides and Krause analyzed the relationship between association and affection measures for Mexican-American children and grandchildren and depression and life satisfaction among the older generation; they found little evidence of a positive association. In fact, high levels of interaction between the generations were significantly related to higher levels of depressive symptoms among the elderly. Mutran and Reitzes (1984) have attributed this perceived dependency in the elderly to be related to high levels of psychological distress. Comparable findings have been observed in families of other ethnic origins, such as Italian Americans (Cohler 1983). Coward (1984) found that older persons who needed some form of assistance had the highest level of life satisfaction if they received it from formal agencies only; those whose sources of assistance consisted largely of informal network support had significantly lower life satisfaction scores. He also found that those who received formal services were not the most disadvantaged or those who had no informal networks to provide assistance.

Why Are Vulnerable Older People Not "Connected" to the System?

Uncomfortable accessing the system. Although there are multiple "system" problems, a very important factor in the at-risk population's failure to access the system lies in the at-risk population's resistance to intervention (Cantor and Mayer 1978). The long-held American belief in rugged individualism tends to reinforce the individual's self-blame for accepting "handouts" when economic and/or health crises occur. An elderly person experiencing physical, emotional, or economic losses may thus attempt to minimize or deny his or her problems and the severity of their impact, because the distress of having to accept his or her need and inability to deal with the problems at hand equal or exceed the pain of the problems themselves. For such a person, asking for assistance would represent an admission of failure too cataclysmic to confront. Feelings of fear, suspicion, shame, and depression lead, almost inevitably, to further isolation and resistance to outside intervention, especially by an agency (Jette and Winnett 1987). The stigma is such that the younger relatives of such a person may also be impacted and thus may discourage or prevent an elder in their family from seeking out or accepting formal services.

Unable to contact services. Community-based agencies continue to expect members of target populations to have sufficient insight, motivation, and resources to access needed services themselves, yet the task of contacting and accessing multiple single-service agencies is difficult for even those who are highly functional and highly motivated (Wylie and Austin 1978). The inability to contact needed services stems from a variety of motivations: some vulnerable elderly, for example, may have difficulties of a practical nature, or minority group members may be unable to speak the language of the service provider and contact persons of the relevant agency.

The elderly person may be too frail or too ill to travel by public transportation yet may have no other means of transportation, owing to poverty or a limited or nonexistent network of persons willing to assist. In others the very nature of the mental and emotional problems from which they suffer renders them incapable of self-referring or accessing needed community care.

Unaware of services available. Last, but certainly not least, the vulnerable elderly may suffer from lack of awareness about the services provided. This lack of awareness can exist at several levels: they may not know any services are available to anyone; they may not know services are available specifically to them; or they may not know that the kind of service they need is available. They may not know that the problem they are facing can be impacted by any service provided. To a vulnerable, isolated elderly individual, little sharing of information is available. This, coupled with the fact that most agencies place the responsibility for learning about and obtaining services squarely on the client, means that many vulnerable elderly do not ask for help because they do not know that any kind of help is available to them. Word of mouth from peers who have successfully interacted with a service-providing agency is often the most trusted and most acceptable means of communicating information about benefits available to needy older clients, yet the relative isolation of the vulnerable older person often blocks this information pathway.

Services are absent or inadequate. It is a sad fact that many vulnerable elderly remain unserved because the services they need are either absent or inadequate. This is particularly obvious in rural areas, for example, where there are no Meals on Wheels programs, no public transportation, no visiting nurses, among others. To the needy older person it matters little whether the service is available but he or she is unable to access it or whether it simply does not exist. The reasons for absent or inadequate services are multiple, ranging from inadequate funding to indifference, but the result is the same: vulnerable older persons remain without access to needed assistance.

Services not geared toward helping a particular client. Many agency programs are planned and executed by white males. The system, like most bureaucracies, is relatively inflexible in many aspects. Thus, the minority client, the ethnically or culturally diverse client, or the client whose lifestyle diverges from that perceived by the mainstream culture to be "normal" or "acceptable" may find it difficult or impossible either to access services or to derive advantages from services offered, once contact has been made.

Caregiver difficulty in dealing with the vulnerable elderly. It may be that formal social service personnel are hiding from the at-risk elderly as often as the elderly are discouraging interaction with them (Harel et al. 1990). Social work and health care practitioners will inevitably experience some of the losses their elderly clients may be currently enduring. Many may wish to avoid confronting a frail client, particularly in a time of crisis, who has been assaulted by repeated losses. Additionally, it is in gerontological practice that professionals are confronted with a person's final destiny; it is impossible, for the caregiver in such a situation, to avoid confrontation with his or her own mortality—a subject with which many, including service providers, are intensely uncomfortable.

Improving the Connection between the Vulnerable Elderly and the "System"

The problems of the vulnerable elderly are such that they demand relief, if not resolution, immediately. Among those who are physically or psychologically weakened, delay can be fatal. In recent decades several hundred federal programs benefitting the elderly either directly or indirectly have been generated, but their apparent abundance serves as no valid indication of their adequacy or their ability to provide service in light of changing social, economic, and demographic conditions related to the aging population. If the vulnerable elderly—long referred to as the "hidden elderly," because of their isolation—are to receive service, they must first be located. Because of reluctance on the part of many such elderly to seek even badly needed services, the person or persons entrusted with locating the vulnerable elderly must elicit their trust. Various avenues can lead to establishing this necessary trust, ranging from simple familiarity with a well-known face, like that of the meter reader or the pharmacist, to the bond of shared experience found with a stranger who also has undergone some of the losses faced by the vulnerable elder.

Securing formal support services for at-risk elderly should be one of the aims of gerontological social work practitioners. Potential provider systems can be harnessed to meet the needs and resources of elderly persons in our society. Untapped resources that can provide the links between the elderly and formal services are community gatekeepers, peers helping peers, informal social support provided by family and friends, and group work intervention empowering individuals to help themselves (see fig. 6).

Community Gatekeepers

Neighborhoods serve as a locus for a number of important social functions, ranging from friendship and sociability, interpersonal influence, and socialization to mutual aid and informal helping (Neparstek et al. 1982). These neighborhood-based ties are especially important to the ethnic elderly. A familiar environment, even if unsafe, contains cues that give the individual a sense of security, continuity, and sameness regarding "person-in-situation." Many elderly persons suffer economic and/or physical limitations; the neighborhood then becomes a highly valuable resource. Older people are more geographically restricted than other groups in the community and are therefore more likely to rely upon neighborhood residents for emotional and social support. To the vulnerable elderly person, buffeted by unasked-for changes and losses, comfort can be found in such simple acts as buying one's daily bread from the same grocer week after week. Buying one's stamps from the same postal clerk or having prescriptions filled by the same pharmacist, time after time, lends a sense of stability to the often extremely precarious world of the elderly individual. The isolated elderly person, in such a situation, is enabled to build a sorely needed sense of alliance: the pharmacy becomes "my pharmacy" and the grocery store "my grocery store." The neighborhood thus lends the individual psychological identification and a sense of commitment—properties much needed by the isolated, vulnerable elderly.

It is possible to enhance the linkage of people to services through the use of community gatekeepers. Gatekeepers are nontraditional referral sources trained

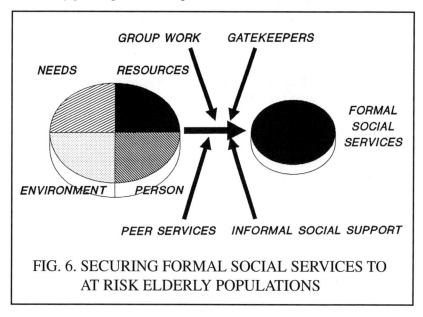

FIG. 6. SECURING FORMAL SOCIAL SERVICES TO
AT RISK ELDERLY POPULATIONS

to identify and locate high-risk elderly in the community (Knight, Reinhart, and Field 1982). The gatekeeper system is composed of nontraditional personnel, such as apartment or mobile home court managers, postal carriers, water meter readers, newspaper carriers, and pharmacists. They are trained to identify and locate vulnerable elderly living in the community who cannot or will not self-refer and who do not have a functional social support network to act on their behalf. Such a community network, enhanced by corporate and other social networks, can alert health and social work professionals to the unmet and undermet needs of their potential client population (Raschko 1991).

Starting in 1987, a program devised jointly by the Virginia Department for the Aging and Virginia Power has linked a gatekeeper to the frail elderly. In this program meter readers are trained to notice such signs of potential problems as piled-up, unread newspapers on the doorstep or in the drive. The gatekeeper alerts the appropriate agency, which can then investigate and initiate service exploration and delivery (Schneider and Kropf 1992).

UTILIZATION OF INFORMAL SOCIAL SUPPORT SYSTEMS

Antonucci (1985) defines social support as interpersonal transactions involving key elements such as aid, affect, or affirmation. In general, it is useful to think of social networks as structures (who or what they are) and social support as functional behaviors (what they do). The combination of social ties—organization memberships, friends, neighbors, and family members—constitute a social network (structure). This collection of interacting, naturally occurring, noninstitutional social relationships meets certain basic social needs of an individual and relates to the individual's adaptation to life's demands (function). Social needs include affection, esteem or approval, sense of belonging, identity, and security, and these needs are met through instrumental supports involving direct tangible assistance or material aid or expressive support involving emotional support and sustenance (Kahn and Antonucci 1980).

Basic to the concept of a social support system is the idea that the assistance provided is a means of augmenting individual competency and mastery over the environment rather than increasing dependency (Cantor 1985). Thus, the helping functions that spring from people's interactions with primary group members in the informal support system lend coherence and well-being to people's lives. For older persons social relationships perceived as satisfying have been likened to a protective cushion against the role losses that are integral to the aging process (Lowenthal and Haven 1968).

Research suggests that older people perceive the informal network of kin, friends, and neighbors as the most appropriate source of social support in most situations of need (Gurian and Cantor 1978). Family and other informal network members are seen by older people as natural extensions of themselves. This emphasis on the family arises from both the family's centrality in providing social care and from its primacy in the lives of the elderly.

In a social network each person has some degree of involvement, and, in the case of family, such reciprocity stretches over the life cycle. Merely having a living spouse, child, or other relative, however, does not guarantee that someone will be willing or able to help in times of crisis. Cantor (1975) introduced the concept of "functional support" in examining the support system of New York City's elderly. In this construct the existence or presence of a support element is not considered sufficient to ensure meaningful assistance. In order for the support element to be considered functional, there must be enough evidence of an ongoing relationship to guarantee meaningful support.

Kahn and Antonucci (1980) employ the highly descriptive term *convoy* to describe the dynamic concept of social networks over the life course:

The individual is surrounded from early childhood by a variety of network members who are sources of social support. Beginning with the well-documented phenomenon of attachment to primary caregivers, the individual develops a variety of interpersonal relationships which become the basis for the support convoy. Many of the members continue and maintain a relationship with the focal person. As the individuals involved grow and mature, the nature of their relationships develops and changes. At different points in the life course, members of the convoy may be lost either through death or less significant changes. At the same time, as the individual matures, and experiences different events and transitions, new convoy members are added.

Thus, according to Kahn and Antonucci, social support networks are in force over the entire life span, but either the structure (network composition) or the participants, or both, may be subject to change. The life span framework of the convoy concept emphasizes the need to examine these exchange patterns over time. Therefore, a person now receiving support may have provided support to others earlier and thus now feels that he or she is drawing from a "support bank" account established long ago (Antonucci 1985).

Parent-child interaction patterns do not generally emerge for the first time in later life. Data suggest (Campbell 1980), rather, that lifelong patterns are present and that these patterns become more evident over time. Thus, it appears especially important among the aged to know the history of a relationship of support exchanges to be able to understand the current nature of the support relationship. This information can enable the service provider more accurately to analyze the actual or potential strengths and weaknesses of an elder person's social network and to determine whether social or health intervention might be necessary.

Antonucci (1988) has also suggested that the norm of reciprocity varies within the context of different relationships and over time. The elderly are more likely to receive support from their children while maintaining reciprocal relationships with their spouses, friends, and neighbors. Wentowski (1981) describes three types of reciprocity: immediate, deferred, and generalized. *Immediate reciprocity* is founded on distance and minimal obligations that can be quickly disposed. In cases of *deferred reciprocity* repayment of a gift or service is postponed, thus encouraging greater trust between the individuals. These two kinds of exchange are both based upon balanced reciprocity, that is, exact repayment. The third type of reciprocity, *generalized reciprocity,* emerges after the first two forms have occurred for some time. In generalized reciprocity exact repayment is no longer expected. The assumption is that persons will contribute to others' well-being and will eventually be compensated themselves. Generalized reciprocity is probably characteristic of the relationship between the elderly and their families.

This interpretation takes into account previous life periods, when older persons provided family members with more support than they received. According to this perspective, it becomes less difficult today for the elderly to maintain relationships in which they receive more than they now provide. The vital balance of reciprocity is maintained, as well as the self-esteem garnered from a sense of having given and provided for others, albeit in the past.

Litwak (1985) provided the conceptual framework that permits classification of the *instrumental* and *affective* components of caregiving. With effectiveness as the desired goal, it is required by Litwak's "balance model of complimentary tasks" that formal organizations handle uniform tasks efficiently and that primary groups, such as families, handle nonuniform tasks humanely. When the system works there is a balance between the efficient and the humane. A partnership between the formal and informal support networks can thus ensure effective care to the older person. Such an alliance is especially valuable to those families whose members are geographically dispersed.

Within American culture the elderly's independence is threatened more by potential reliance on kin than reliance on government services. The elderly are undoubtedly grateful for the affection and expressive support shown them by their families; however, it does not follow that they will be pleased to take advantage of these sentiments. Kin are the natural link to the social support system of the elderly. Nevertheless, acknowledging the geographic distances between family members, the demands on their time, and mushrooming financial costs, dependence on the formal support system for uniform tasks will guarantee an equilibrium of care.

The existence of functional social support has been blamed for nonparticipation by the older adult in formal social service programs. In actuality, the support of the informal helping network has been found to be the best predictor of social service use by rural elderly (Goodfellow 1983).

The current focus within social work practice theories upon the individual's transactions with the social environment as the point of intervention for social workers makes a fuller, more precise understanding and use of informal support networks important to the effectiveness of the profession. Awareness that there may be important variation in the nature of social support among different kinds of kin relationships and that kin relationships are not always present in the informal social networks of some elderly individuals should prompt social workers to prepare more differential assessment and intervention plans.

For many older adults, particularly those previously defined as the vulnerable elderly, friends and neighbors form the only informal support network available. Recognition of the importance of such bonds, and of the possibility for both expressive and tangible help arising from such relationships, should alert professional community practitioners to the possibility of new sources of informal support in clients.

Peer Services

Like informal support systems, peer services represent another resource for community practitioners. Peer services for older persons have enjoyed great popularity and apparent success, as exemplified by programs such as the national Retired Senior Volunteer Program. It is not difficult to understand the underlying basis for this positive response. To peer service providers such programs offer an important social role to replace roles lost because of retirement and the deaths of friends and significant others. For older individuals in need of services it is often less demeaning to receive services from one's peers than from members of the younger generation. A peer is less likely to be made uneasy, even repelled, by the often unpleasant physical and/or mental changes that can accompany old age, and this greater comfort with the situation promotes greater acceptance on the part of both the care provider and care recipient. Retirees are, in brief, a vast and untapped resource who are perhaps the best equipped of all to assist their fellow elderly (Kahn 1973).

Anne Eaton founded the Life Enrichment Services (LES), a nonprofit group that helps older people help one another. With no government money, but with some forty thousand volunteer hours each year, LES provides older people in Atlanta, Georgia, with useful services such as a widowed persons' service, which provides peer counseling and teaches survival skills, and a semivolunteer older "handyman corps" that provides inexpensive home repairs. This self-help community senior organization is an example from among hundreds of similar enterprises that have been established across the country, capitalizing on the skills and energy of the well elderly to help other older persons and help link them up with established health and social services.

Some corporations (e.g., Wells Fargo) have recruited retired senior volunteers to help local nonprofit agencies. Blue Cross and Blue Shield of Indiana has hired retired people with backgrounds in insurance, accounting, or teaching to explain the confusing interaction between Medicare and private insurance policies to older homebound, often bedridden, subscribers. Members of this Blue Cross and Blue Shield "Ambassador Corps" take pride in their work, because it keeps them busy in a productive way, and they enjoy the respect and satisfaction they garner from helping their peers. The consumers appreciate the personal attention, along with the financial savings achieved through wiser money management (Dychtwald 1990).

Dychtwald (1990) has also suggested other volunteer peer services that can be of benefit, both to peer providers and service recipients, including the use of health care advocates and group services.

Health Care Advocates

Retired doctors, nurses, and other health professionals could be available in physicians' offices and hospitals to help patients fill out forms and to answer their questions about Medicare, patients' rights, and social services, among others.

Group Services

Group services represent another referral source for community practioners. The loss of a spouse and/or significant others leaves an older person alone, surrounded by a world of the past. The loneliness and deprivation of surviving loved ones engenders a sense of irrelevance and status anxiety unknown to the majority of younger people but very familiar to an older person's peers. In order to achieve reconnection with what is now an altered and unfamiliar world and in order to adapt personal identity and role to accommodate the changes,

133

the elderly need to share their thoughts, feelings, and past and present experiences with a cohort who understands and can validate their existence. Participation in a meaningful group provides the older person with vital emotional support and commonality of experiences. The pain of grief and loss can often be ameliorated enormously just by the testimony of others that affirms for the person "I am not the only person who has experienced such a loss, and I am not the only person who has felt the way I feel right now."

Perhaps even more important is that participation in a group enables the elderly person to develop a reciprocal relationship with peers which allows him or her to be a giver as well as a recipient of both emotional and tangible support. The opportunity to contribute empowers the elderly, building badly needed self-esteem and sense of self-worth. The loss of significant others in one's life is often marked less by the sense of what one no longer is able to receive from the missing person than by the fact that one can no longer contribute to the missing individual and, subsequently, receive validation from him or her. Being able, once again, to contribute something to others is ego supportive and, therefore, a highly effective antidote to depression. According to Lowy (1983), "Group associations can provide many opportunities to replace old friends with new ones, to substitute family ties with peer ties, and to give new status and hence new relevance to one's existence."

Groups can also serve as information resources and translators concerning available services. Hirayama (1983) has written of the utility of group work with minority elderly: "Information related to the availability of services and how and what to do to obtain them may be dispensed in groups. Misconceptions about eligibilities and value conflicts and resistance to approaching agencies may be resolved in group processes. Importantly, facilitation of a mutual aid system among members encourages their individual self-determination." In persons experiencing difficulty accessing formal services, whether because of ethnic or cultural differences or because of individual reluctance to seek or accept help, shared experiences within the group can provide needed information, clear up misunderstandings, and bolster the confidence of the reluctant, so that they are able to apply for and accept needed assistance.

Learned helplessness is a by-product of our current social service and health care delivery system, which is most often based on individual means tests and is characterized by inadequacies, bureaucratic red tape, and stigmatization, which compound the development of a sense of powerlessness. Powerlessness is also reinforced by the social and psychological pressures attached to persistent ageist attitudes in the United States. For the frail elderly who have had a lifetime of experience providing for themselves and their families and who are, through the physical and mental onslaughts of aging, losing control over themselves and their lives, it is extremely difficult to turn to services that are totally out of their control. It is a basic fact of human existence that much of our fortune depends upon society at large and also upon the support of those close to us. The logical extension of this interdependency would be to turn to the formal network of services provided by the society in which we live. Yet the stigma attached by the current system to accepting care and the historical American legacy of rugged individualism make many elderly extremely reluctant to apply for and accept even badly needed assistance, whereas in other developed countries such services would be regarded by the elderly as something they had earned by being productive members of society during their working lifetimes. Group support can transmit the important message: "This is what you need, this is how you get it, and it is OK to take it," thus connecting the vulnerable elderly to the formal support system and providing the valuable psychological support they need to accept needed support and retain their self-esteem.

Although collective resources fall far short of meeting existing needs, service recipients have not organized to demand that access and delivery be improved; this lack of group participation has reinforced alienation, a major component of learned helplessness (Cox 1989). Group-oriented empowerment interventions make the important connection between working with individuals and working for social change. Cox and Longres (1981) stress the importance of the "personal as political" as a key element of intervention. Even though the orientation is focused on the group, each individual in the group is engaging in an authentic struggle for personal survival and improvement of his or her own environment. The individual group participant accrues benefits ranging from enhanced productivity, psychological well-being, attainment of a role, and possible status attached to that role as well as a core of group members upon whom he or she can rely for acceptance and even possible assistance. These benefits, which group members of any age can attain, are especially vital to the elderly, among whom feelings of irrelevance and uselessness, by-products of role losses and isolation, must be combated in order to maintain the psychological well-being of the elderly person beset by ongoing, progressive losses.

Once engaged, many elderly begin to consider themselves as part of a more promising alternative. As part of a collective experience in social change, they once again experience the self-empowerment produced by having self-determination. Part of this empowerment process is provided by linking an individual's personal struggles with his or her environment, his or her community, and, ultimately, to the society, as a whole, in which he or she lives. Group work can thus transform personal problems into consciousness-raising issues and social policy change (Cox 1989) and, through this expanded perspective, provide the "reconnection" that those who are isolated and alienated so desperately need and, most often, are unable to find on their own.

The particular focus of the group, whether it be concerned, for example, with alternative housing and home sharing skills or the improvement of health-related communications, is not of primary importance. What is vital is that the group experience provide an education in personal and group consciousness for the participants which translates into social change for them and for the greater good of society. The vulnerable elderly, whom we have previously discussed, frequently have no network of kin and suffer feelings of profound worthlessness for a variety of reasons, some personal and some societal. Even a first visit to a group is likely to dispel some of the feelings of isolation; a vulnerable older person feels, "I am not completely alone." Further investigation and group participation and sharing will extend this observation: "I am not the only one who feels as I do." This recognition of shared humanity forms a powerful antidote to feelings of personal unworthiness and self-rejection. Further identification of the causes of the individual's problems will likely lead to recognition of some of them and an understanding that aspects of the problems do not lie solely with the individual. At this point an appreciation of the possibility for change enters the picture. The individual realizes that, just as his or her individual problems form part of a larger, collective problem, so his or her participation in the group can make a contribution to a larger, collective solution, which, as an individual, he or she could not make. This recognition, that the power of the group is greater than the sum of the power of the various individual members, and the fact that the individual is personally enhanced by being part of this endeavor create a basis for a powerful link between the once isolated individual and the world outside—a link that can form the basis for potent, life-enriching change, both within the individual and in society at large.

In our society vast numbers of the hidden elderly live out their final days in loneliness and depression, tormented by feelings of worthlessness and irrelevance, themselves often exacerbated by guilt over having such feelings. Some have no family; some have family members who have turned away from them; some have family members, but they are too distant to provide needed help; and some live in the isolation of rural areas. Formal assistance is available at varying levels, but many of the vulnerable elderly do not access the benefits to which they are entitled. Some believe that to do so would be an admission of personal failure, some do not know that assistance is available for their particular problem(s), and some have no knowledge that benefits of any kind are available.

In a time when maximization of resources is the watchword, surely maximization of human resources should represent a societal imperative. Linkage to formal services is, for many, particularly the vulnerable elderly, a lifeline to an enhanced quality of life in the latter years. Independent community practitioners can use informal and formal support systems to supplement their own activities.

REFERENCES

Antonucci, T. (1985). Personal characteristics, social support, and social behavior. In *Handbook of aging and the social sciences,* ed. R. Binstock and E. Shanas, 2d ed., 94–119. New York: Van Nostrand Reinhold.
———. (1988). Reciprocal and nonreciprocal social support: Contrasting sides of intimate relationships. *Journal of Gerontology* 43, no. 3: S65–73.
Broderick, A. (1988). Hawaii's Filipino elderly: Underutilization of social services. MS, Honolulu.
Campbell, A. (1980). *A sense of well-being in America.* New York: McGraw-Hill.
Cantor, M. H. (1975). Life space and the social support system of the inner-city elderly of New York. *Gerontologist* 15:23–27.
———. (1985). Aging and social care. In *Handbook of aging and the social sciences,* ed. R. Binstock and E. Shanas, 2d ed., 745–81. New York: Van Nostrand Reinhold.
Cantor, M. H., and M. J. Mayer. (1978). Factors in differential utilization of services by urban elderly. *Journal of Gerontological Social Work* 1:47–61.
Cath, S. (1963). Some dynamics of the middle and later years. *Smith College Studies in Social Work* 33, no. 2: 174–90.
Cohler, B. (1983). Autonomy and interdependence in the family of adulthood: A psychological perspective. *Gerontologist* 23:33–39.
Coward, R. T. (1984). The helping network of noninstitutionalized elders: Changes in the mixture of formal and informal helpers. Committee on Studies of Aging, McGill University, Montreal.
Cox, E. O. (1989). Empowerment of low income elderly through group work. In *Group work with the poor and oppressed,* ed. E. O. Cox, 111–25. New York: Haworth Press.
Cox, E. O., and J. Longres. (1981). Critical practice-curriculum implications. Annual meeting of the Council of Social Work Education, Louisville, Ky.
Cuellar, J. B., and J. Weeks. (1980). Minority elderly Americans: A profile

for area agencies on aging—executive summary. Administration on Aging (AOA) grant 90-A-1667, Allied Home Health Association. San Diego, Calif.: Author.

Dychtwald, K. (1990). *Age wave.* New York: Bantam Books.

Gelfand, D., and C. Barresi, eds. (1987). *Ethnic dimensions of aging.* New York: Springer.

Germain, C. B., ed. (1979). *Social work practice: People and environments.* New York: Columbia University Press.

Goodfellow, M. (1983). Reasons for use and nonuse of social services among the rural elderly. *Human Services in the Rural Environment* 8, no. 4: 10–16.

Gurian, B., and M. H. Cantor. (1978). Mental health and community support systems for the elderly. In *Aging: The process and the people,* ed. G. Usdin, and C. Hofling, 184–205. New York: Brunner/Mazel.

Harel, Z., P. Ehrlich, and R. Hubbard. (1990). *The vulnerable aged: People, services, and policies.* New York: Springer.

Hendricks, K., and C. D. Hendricks. (1986). *Aging in mass society.* Boston: Little, Brown.

Hepworth, D. H., and J. Larsen. (1993). *Direct social work protocol.* Pacific Grove, Calif.: Cole.

Hirayama, H. (1983). Group services for the minority aged. In *Aging in minority groups,* ed. R. L. McNeely and J. L. Colen. Beverly Hills, Calif.: Sage, 270–80.

Jette, C. B., and R. L. Winnett. (1987). Late-onset paranoid disorder. *American Journal of Orthopsychiatry* 57:485–94.

Kahn, A. J. (1973). *Social policy and social services.* New York: Random House.

Kahn, R. L., and T. Antonucci. (1980). Convoys over the life course: Attachment role and social support. In *Lifespan development and behavior,* ed. P. B. Baltes and O. G. Brim, 254–83. New York: Academic Press.

Knight, B., R. Reinhart, and P. Field. (1982). Senior outreach services: A treatment-oriented outreach team in community mental health. *Gerontologist* 22:544–47.

Litwak, E. (1985). *Helping the elderly: The complementary roles of informal networks and formal systems.* New York: Guilford Press.

Lowenthal, M. F., and C. Haven. (1968). Interaction and adaptation: Intimacy as a critical variable. *American Sociological Review* 33:20–30.

Lowy, L. (1983). Social group work with vulnerable older persons: A theoretical perspective. *Social Work with Groups* 5, no. 2: 21–32.

138

Markides, K. S., and N. Krause. (1985). Intergenerational solidarity and psychological well-being among older Mexican Americans: A three generations study. *Journal of Gerontology* 40:390–92.

Markides, K. S., and C. Mindel. (1987). *Aging and ethnicity.* Beverly Hills, Calif.: Sage.

Mutran, E., and D. C. Reitzes. (1984). Intergenerational support activities and well-being among the elderly: A convergence of exchange and symbolic interaction perspectives. *American Sociological Review* 49:117–39.

Neparstek, A., D. Biegel, and H. Spiro. (1982). *Neighborhood networks for humane mental health care.* New York: Plenum.

Raschko, R. (1991). *Gatekeeper training manual.* Spokane, Wash.: Spokane Community Mental Health Center.

Rosenfeld, J. (1983). The domain and expertise of social work: A conceptualization. *Social Work* 28:186–91.

Scheidt, R. A. (1984). Taxonomy of well-being for small-town elderly: A case for rural diversity. *Gerontologist* 24:84–90.

Schneider, L., and N. P. Kropf. (1992). *Gerontological social work.* Chicago: Nelson-Hall.

Wentowski, G. J. (1981). Reciprocity and the coping strategies of older people: Cultural dimensions of network building. *Gerontologist* 21:600–609.

Wylie, M., and C. Austin. (1978). Policy foundations for case management: Consequences for the frail elderly. *Journal of Gerontological Social Work* 1:7–17.

Chapter 9

THE ROLE OF COMMUNITY PRACTITIONERS
The Service Network

This chapter focuses on describing the cast of practitioners involved in community service to the elderly and their specific roles and responsibilities. The medical profession traditionally has provided the standard for independent, or solo, practice in health care. Although that standard has been brought under close scrutiny due to growing interest in cost containment and preventive health care, a model of independent private practice still has merit and, metaphorically speaking, should not be "thrown out with the bathwater." It is, however, incumbent upon professionals to become more responsible in terms of regulating their own practices and seeing to it that their clients or patients receive the advantages that comprehensive screening and coordinated care can provide. The remainder of the book is devoted to defining the professional roles and the range of professionals with whom the older person is likely to have contact. Their mutual responsibility to identify the scope of an individual's service needs and to make appropriate referrals will also be discussed. This last component of practice is not a formally institutionalized function of many professions. Nursing, social work, and public health incorporate a broad range of responsibility within the scope of professional responsibility, including an emphasis on service coordination. Medical doctors, on the other hand, have been slow to recognize their role in prevention and chronic care management and prefer to work autonomously. Although interdisciplinary practice is a hallmark of hospital and nursing home care provision, community service tends to be fragmented. Managed-care organizations, for example, health maintenance organizations, have been more effective in instituting cost constraints than in meeting their alleged objective of promoting wellness through preventive health care. The present chapter begins with a description of the activities of the various community practitioners and concludes with the specifics of their responsibilities for screening and referral.

GERIATRICIANS

A geriatrician, or geriatric medical doctor, is a physician who has specialized in the management of the health problems of older adults. As with any specialist, a geriatrician has the highest level of expertise in the management of the health requirements of the elderly. The geriatrician, like the specialist in family practice, is involved in the treatment of the whole person and incorporates a focus on preventive maintenance. Geriatric medicine currently is not among the more popular medical fields, in part as a result of reimbursement limitations under Medicare. House calls used to be a routine activity for geriatricians; however, restrictions on reimbursement and a growing demand for service have driven most geriatricians to limit their practices to the office. The geriatrician generally is not the patient's primary physician. Most older people have internists, from whom they receive primary care. If the internist is the primary-care physician, the internist should utilize the resources of the geriatric consultant, as he or she would utilize any other specialist. The internist then becomes the one responsible for integrating a coordinated care plan and making appropriate referrals. The methodology of coordination is spelled out in the next chapter.

GEROPSYCHIATRISTS AND GEROPSYCHOTHERAPISTS

A regulatory pitfall that plagues the mental health arena is the lack of regulation. Anyone can call him- or herself a psychotherapist. Similarly, anyone who does psychotherapy with the elderly can call him- or herself a geropsychotherapist. The area in which psychotherapy is regulated is in the process of certification for reimbursement under private insurers and Medicare or Medicaid. In the state of New York, for example, only three types of mental health professionals are certified to receive insurance reimbursement: psychiatrists, advanced-degree clinical psychologists (Ph.D. or Psy.D.), and social workers with at least a master's degree in social work (M.S.W.).

Geropsychiatrists need very little explaining. They are licensed medical doctors specializing in geropsychiatry, or the diagnosis and treatment of the mental health problems associated with aging. Geropsychotherapists typically are geriatric social workers, geriatric psychologists, or geropsychiatric nurses. Among these social workers, psychologists, and nurses the commonalities in

141

approach may outweigh the differences; nevertheless, it is useful to delineate some of their differences. Social work training emphasizes individual people in specific situations and incorporates a consideration of psychological and social influences (e.g., the family or social status) upon a person's mental health. Many social workers practice in outpatient mental health clinics, family counseling agencies, or inpatient hospitals.

Private practice has always provided an alternative arena for social workers. The clinical psychologist's education and training emphasize the diagnosis and treatment of mental illness as well as attention to psychological and neurological predeterminants. The psychiatric nurse's training is in the management of psychiatric illness. Most nurses practice in mental health clinics and hospital systems and their education incorporates an emphasis that includes biological, psychological, and social aspects of mental disease. Nursing practice reflects the medical model of study, diagnosis, and treatment. Assessment and continuity of care planning are integral aspects of nursing practice.

The geropsychiatrist is the only professional among those mentioned who traditionally has prescribed medication. In some states nurse practitioners are currently licensed to prescribe certain medications. The clinical psychologist generally is the one to perform intelligence or mental status testing. The social worker traditionally includes within the scope of his or her tasks a focus on mediating the needs of the client and the demands of the client's support system—for example, family, job, health agency, social service agency, or house of worship.

Although there are certain ideological differences in orientation among these different mental health professionals, what really distinguishes one professional from another is his or her postgraduate training and experience. Some geropsychiatrists and some geropsychotherapists have received psychoanalytic or advanced clinical training, and others have not. Clinical training is the key to understanding differences in treatment methodology. Some therapists are behaviorists and emphasize the need to monitor and change behavior; other approaches are more humanistic, emphasizing concern about the person rather than his or her symptoms. There are many possible variations on the roles played by these mental health practitioners. If, however, a mental health practitioner chooses to specialize in the problems of aging, it is essential that at least two criteria are met: the geropsychotherapist must receive training about treating the special mental health problems of the elderly and must be committed to a comprehensive treatment approach focusing on the biological, social, legal, financial, and spiritual realities of his or her clients or patients.

THE GERIATRIC CASE MANAGER

The geriatric case manager is a relatively new professional designation. Case managers are usually private organizations or practitioners and include social workers, registered nurses, and other types of human service professionals. The primary responsibility of the case manager is comprehensive assessment and coordination of appropriate long-term care services. The geriatric case manager is not a state-licensed position. There are no regulatory requirements for case managers other than those associated with the licensed profession with which they are involved—for example, social work or nursing. A case manager's particular expertise also derives from his or her professional background. The common denominator for geriatric case management is a focus on resource coordination.

THE ELDER LAWYER

Elder law describes the activities of attorneys who specialize in providing service to older people. These legal services include counseling individuals in the following areas: eligibility for nursing home coverage; eligibility for home care coverage; eligibility for Medicare, Medicaid, Social Security, Disability, Worker's Compensation; the transfer of assets and spousal responsibility for meeting health care costs; hospital discharge policies; preretirement financial planning; estate planning; and planning for incapacity. Although no special licensure is required to practice elder law, attorneys choosing this area of practice must take a comprehensive view of their elder clients' legal and financial needs. They also should be prepared to "network" with other human service professionals. As with the medical field, a client's primary attorney may regard him- or herself not as an elder rights specialist but, rather, as a general practitioner. This does not clear an attorney of any ethical responsibility to provide a comprehensive legal service to his or her client or to make the appropriate referral to a specialist in elder law.

THE GERIATRIC FINANCIAL ADVISOR

Financial advisors run the gamut from certified public accountants to financial planners. The designation is a catchall for professionals who are primarily concerned with the financial issues related to aging, such as preretirement planning, estate planning, planning for incapacity, tax preparation, and insurance coverage. Financial concerns frequently serve as a more critical impetus for one's seeking help than medical or social problems. A financial advisor may be the first line of defense in making a comprehensive assessment and managing related medical or social problems.

143

RELIGIOUS LEADERS

Many people become more involved with regard to religion as they age. The older individual's lack of church or synagogue attendance is attributed to transportation and mobility difficulties, not lack of spirituality or motivation. The priest, nun, minister, or rabbi might also be the first individual a person in need will turn to, particularly in a time of loss and bereavement. Sometimes spiritual counsel is sufficient to stem a wave of emotional or physical decline; other times an individual may need help of a secular nature. Nuns are highly involved in the social activities of their parishioners. They frequently participate on interagency planning committees and councils. Their contribution to the community, though unheralded, is of immense significance.

Religious connections generally are not foremost in the minds of other human service professionals, such as nurses and social workers. It is essential that the clergy as well as all human service professionals recognize one another's importance to the health and welfare of their clients, patients, and congregants.

GERIATRIC NURSES

Geriatric nurses specialize in the health care needs of older people. There are many kinds of nurses, including public health nurses and nurse practitioners. A nurse's formal educational background and clinical training influence his or her role orientation. Public health nursing, for example, emphasizes prevention and community education. Traditional hospital-based nursing has always focused more on physical diagnosis and assisting physicians in the implementation of medical treatment plans. The nurse practitioner is licensed in some states to practice independently and to prescribe certain medications. Nursing has always recognized the importance of comprehensive assessment. In recent years turf battles with social workers in hospitals have been waged over which profession should have control over discharge planning and continuity of care planning. Different resolutions have been worked out in various facilities, but for both professions case management has assumed a more central role. This bodes well for patients, who will benefit from more integrated care planning. The community nurse is most likely going to be working for a home care agency or in public health. Organizations are accustomed to dealing with other agencies, such as hospitals and social service agencies. The approach being presented here suggests that agency personnel and private practitioners must coordinate their activities.

144

GERIATRIC NUTRITIONISTS

The importance of diet in maintaining good health has achieved widespread recognition. Most nutritionists practice within an agency framework, such as a hospital, school, or clinic. The management of good nutrition, however, is part of a broad-sweeping trend toward wellness in health promotion; thus, a growing number of nutritionists practice independently or in the private sector. They are also used as consultants to businesses that market health foods, dietary supplements, or diet and exercise plans. Nutritionists will join the host of other physical fitness professionals who are becoming more and more central to the lives of all Americans. The nutritionist is another link in the service continuum.

SCREENING AND REFERRAL

Each professional is responsible for screening and proper referral. The following highlight the types of issues that should serve as trigger mechanisms requiring professionals to refer their clients or patients to those from other disciplines. Reasons for referral are obviously not limited to these issues.

Screening Triggers for the Geriatrician

The geriatrician, or medical doctor for the elderly, is responsible for managing the chronic care needs of his or her patients and promoting wellness. The primary reason people seek medical care is that they perceive they have a problem; they are either physically symptomatic, hypochondriacal, or do not know what professional to utilize. In traditional American medicine wellness and prevention have not been emphasized. Therefore, the reliance on symptoms as an impetus to seeking medical attention largely is a function of indoctrination.

Older people have to be reeducated to seek routine medical or nursing care. Nevertheless, most will require treatment for one or more of the various chronic conditions typical of older adults, such as hypertension, heart disease, arthritis, depression, and cognitive dysfunction. The medical doctor must be on the alert for potential complications of polypharmacy and for psychological concomitants of medical conditions. The anguish of coping with physical limitations can be expected to have a negative impact on one's mental health. In addition, financial concerns or legal questions can create significant stress, which might exacerbate the symptoms of any physical condition. Family conflicts are apt to arise when tensions over failing health or confusion over treatment options mount. The connections between diet, exercise, lifestyle factors (e.g., sexual behavior or leisure activity), and physical and mental health cannot be underestimated. The medical doctor must be on the alert for all possible connections

145

Screening Triggers* for Different Professionals

PROFESSION	PRIMARY FOCUS	TRIGGERS
Geriatrician	Medical assessment and treatment	Stress related to physical distance; polypharmacy; diet/exercise; lifestyle; family conflicts
Geropsychiatrist/ Geropsychotherapist	"Bio-psycho-social" assessment; biopsychiatric treatment; psychotherapy	Planning for incapacity; resource coordination; physical losses
Case manager	Resource coordination	Psychological stresses; legal issues; financial issues; physical losses
Elder lawyer	Estate planning; planning for incapacity; application for benefits	Family conflicts; elder abuse; physical frailty
Financial advisor	Retirement planning; tax preparation; insurance	Legal issues; psychological stresses
Religious leader	Spiritual counsel	Bereavement; extended illness
Geriatric nurse	Home care	Caregiving issues; physical change; mental change; financial change
Nutritionist	Dietary instruction	Physical health; lifestyle

*triggers represent common problems associated with use of particular service that suggest the need for collateral contacts and evaluate the health consequences. A careful screening, utilizing the Multidisciplinary Screening Instrument described in the next chapter (and given in full in the appendix), will ensure the potential for the appropriate intervention and outcome.

SCREENING TRIGGERS FOR THE GEROPSYCHIATRIST AND GEROPSYCHOTHERAPIST

The older client or patient will not necessarily freely seek the services of either the geropsychiatrist or geropsychotherapist. As the next generation of older adults comes of age, however, there should be a greater openness to psychotherapy among these future older-age cohorts because society has changed its views about psychological health. Typically, if an older person seeks psychotherapy, the prevailing reason will be some type of life adjustment, such as retirement or the sickness or death of a spouse. Geropsychotherapists must be on the alert for signs of diminished physical health, which is often exacerbated by stress. Coordination with a geropsychiatrist is fairly routine for many psychotherapists, who recognize the importance of biopsychiatric assessment and offering possible relief with correct psychopharmacology.

The geropsychotherapist should recognize the social context of the client's or patient's presenting mental disturbance. Often there is a need to involve a lawyer about planning for incapacity and issues regarding health care decision making. If there is a need for resource coordination and the psychotherapist does not view this as an appropriate part of his or her role, then referral to a geriatric case manager is indicated. This professional can assist with long-term care planning or applying for health care benefits.

Screening Triggers for the Geriatric Case Manager

The geriatric care manager has to be most careful in defining the scope of his or her responsibilities. Utilizing the services of other human service professionals may be appropriate. Geriatric case managers who are social workers or psychiatric nurses are accustomed to dealing with the emotional issues that often arise in long-term planning. Other professionals who act as care managers may need to consult with a mental health professional, for example, a psychiatrist, social worker, or psychologist. Comprehensive screening of the patient's needs is viewed here as being essential to any kind of task-focused work. Most long-term care planning involves legal and financial aspects, which require referral to the appropriate professional.

147

Screening Triggers for the Elder Lawyer

It is inevitable that the elder lawyer will interface with many other human service professionals in performing his or her legal activities. Some screening triggers are more subtle than others. For example, estate planning can be very stressful, and frequently individuals will delay the completion of a will because of their own indecision or family conflict. Additionally, older clients may be more vulnerable to abuse than younger ones, because of their perceived or actual increased dependence upon their children or other relatives. Elder lawyers must be attuned to the potential for financial or psychological abuse and be prepared to mediate conflicts or offer protection to their elderly clients. Consultation with a geropsychotherapist may be beneficial in identifying the interests of an elder client and resolving family disputes.

Another, less subtle example of the type of legal problem which suggests the need for consultation with other professionals regards the area of health care decision making or planning for incapacity. A family in which an elder parent has been diagnosed with a physically or mentally degenerative condition will need emotional support and help with continuity of care planning; for example, a referral to nursing home, hospice, or respite program may be essential. The lawyer may choose to work with a geriatric nurse, social worker, or case manager in coordinating resources. Many older people have undiagnosed medical conditions or suffer nutritional deficits or the effects of polypharmacy abuse. These types of health problems can result in reversible cognitive impairment or depression. Any patient or client who displays a symptom of mental disorder should be evaluated to determine its physical cause. A geropsychiatrist's services can be very useful in separating biological and psychological factors and coordinating medical treatment.

The elder lawyer may be the one to whom the older person turns for assistance with financial management, for example, tax preparation or referral to Social Security. The attorney may choose to work with a financial planner in identifying and ensuring the client's financial security throughout retirement.

Screening Triggers for the Geriatric Financial Advisor

The geriatric financial advisor is a relatively new addition to the array of professionals who provide service to the elderly in the community. Geriatric financial advisors are basically responsible for managing their clients' money. The accountability of these professionals is related to the nature of the bond that exists between them and their clients. Clients place their faith in their financial advisors and expect to have their welfare placed above that person's self-interest. Although, traditionally, those in the world of business do not formally network with health professionals, there is a link between financial concerns and legal and health risks. Sometimes it is a concern with failing health which prompts an individual to seek financial advice. The signing of a durable power of attorney can avoid much unnecessary complication if the client should no longer be able to meet the demands of managing his or her own financial responsibilities. The desirability of seeking legal consultation is obvious in this situation, as in others, in which, for example, the transfer of assets may be required for eligibility for Medicaid. An individual's health may suffer because of stresses related to financial worries or insecurities. At such times it may be appropriate for the advisor to recommend medical or psychological counseling. Perhaps it is more of a challenge for nonhealth professionals than health professionals to incorporate an understanding of the needs of the whole person into their sense of professional purpose. It is, nevertheless, equally as critical in ensuring the client's health and well-being.

Screening Triggers for Religious Leaders

Religious leaders have a particularly strong influence over the minds and hearts of older people because of increased spirituality among the elderly. Furthermore, the church pew holds more meaning than the psychoanalyst's couch for people over sixty-five today, who traditionally have sought religious consolation, in contrast to psychotherapy, during periods of stress. Though religion may be more important to older people and particularly to current older-age cohorts, religious attendance often is jeopardized by physical frailty and the lack of transportation. Religious leaders can and do serve as important allies to other human service professionals; however, their role as vital members of the multidisciplinary network needs clarification. Religious leaders are likely to be called upon in times of bereavement or extended illness. They can and should be available for spiritual consolation and guidance. Just as in hospitals, in which the centrality of religious worship to the patient's progress has long been acknowledged and ensured, through the participation of the clergy in interdisciplinary team meetings, religious consultation has its place in community service. While religious leaders are identifying new ways to reach their homebound congregants, other human service providers need to recognize when consultation with clergy is more appropriate than with secular mental health professionals. This is where knowledge of the importance of religion or prayer to an individual is crucial in determining his or her need for religious connection.

Screening Triggers for Geriatric Nurses

The nurse or nurse's aide is probably the most likely individual to be monitoring an old person's health progress, since it is the very old individual (over eighty) who is likely to be receiving services of a home health care agency. Medical and health treatment is better ensured by the involvement of a home care agency; the geriatric nurse, however, is in an ideal position to identify potential cases of mental or physical abuse. Similarly, the nurse should be on the alert for changes in the psychological status of homebound or physically compromised individuals and for potential family conflicts surrounding caregiving. Otherwise, geriatric nurses, like physicians, should understand the connections between such factors as nutrition, exercise, recreation, financial security, protection of personal liberties, and peace of mind in promoting health and should arrange for referrals to community agencies or private practitioners for required services.

Screening Triggers for the Geriatric Nutritionist

Diet is critical in maintaining good health and promoting longevity. Although nutritionists generally work in health clinics, in which patients will have been referred to them for dietary instruction, an astute nutritionist can detect dietary high-risk factors, such as obesity, high cholesterol, too few vitamins, low calcium, and the disease possibilities with which deficiencies are associated and, consequently, help to clarify a patient's condition. The geriatric nutritionist is just one of many allied or ancillary health professionals with whom the elderly may have contact. Pharmacists, physical therapists, dentists, podiatrists, chiropractors, speech therapists, and audiologists all may have an opportunity to screen for related medical, psychological, and social problems. The pharmacist, for example, must be alert to the presentation of side effects or harmful results of drug interactions. The point is that all professionals need to adopt a comprehensive view of the elderly patient because of the interrelationship of health, mental health, spiritual, and social influences upon the patient's welfare. The past practice of intraprofessional collegial activity must be replaced by a new standard of interprofessional collegial activity if the older person's needs are to be met.

This chapter has described the types of professionals who represent the multidisciplinary network in community elder practice, including the geriatrician, geropsychotherapist, elder lawyer, financial advisor, case manager, religious leader, nurse, nutritionist, and other allied and ancillary health professionals. Generic titles such as geropsychotherapist were used, instead of

150

more traditional professional classifications such as psychologist or social worker. Traditional professional titles may be subsumed under broader rubrics, such as geropsychotherapist or geriatric case manager, and are differentiated according to professional task or function. In other words, the authors do not incorporate standard professional distinctions in classifying individual practitioners. Classification is based on practical considerations, depending upon the primary focus of the practitioner's service objectives. The categories reflect the overlap in professional roles among disciplines. The authors employ empirical classification to encourage practitioners to define the range and limits of their professional interventions. The message being communicated is: it is important to know where one's role begins and ends in evaluating the need for collateral contacts with other professionals.

This chapter has also emphasized the high-risk factors that might manifest themselves in various practice arenas. Each practitioner is encouraged to be on the alert for signals that might trigger the need for a referral to another human service professional. These screening triggers represent the variety of presenting problems that provide warning of the potential need for multidisciplinary assessment and intervention.

Chapter 10

ELDER ASSESSMENT
A Multidisciplinary Approach

Given the rapidly expanding elderly population and the resulting need for existing services to be delivered in the most effective, efficient manner possible, careful and accurate assessment of the elderly and their problems and needs has assumed a whole new sense of urgency and importance.

Effective problem solving by carefully analyzing a problem and thoughtfully tailoring a solution is hardly a new concept. Why, then, does this issue deserve special attention in regard to delivery of services to the elderly? In what way is the situation of the elderly unique? The answer to this question lies in both the aging individual as a person and in the nature of the aging process itself. Both components must be carefully studied and analyzed, and the nature of the vast number of variables must be confronted.

OLDER ADULTS ARE INDIVIDUALS

Older adults are possibly the most diverse group of clients with whom social, legal, and health care providers will practice and interact. Clearly, older adults, as a group, appear to be at greater risk than younger people, because of the general vicissitudes of life in the older adult years; however, preventive, restorative, and continuing care interventions cannot be designed or carried out in any effective manner without carefully considering the lack of heterogeneity among this segment of the population. Contrary to prevailing myths, older adults probably differ more from one another than do the individuals of any other age group.

Ethnic and cultural differences. The minority elderly represent a diverse group of individuals. Their language, styles of interpersonal relating, and viewpoints toward social, health, and other services are often at variance from those of the mainstream culture. Adherence to these cultural mores can represent stability and security to the minority elderly; therefore, individual ethnic and cultural differences must be carefully taken into account when assessing a problem and attempting to devise a solution.

Economic differences. Many of the elderly seeking services are poor. On the other hand, the wide availability of Social Security to today's elderly has provided increased independence to this group of people. People who have been poor all their lives may have found a way to live effective, meaningful lives within the confines of their economic limitations, or they may have suffered depression and loss of self-esteem as the result of chronic poverty. Persons who have enjoyed relative prosperity so long as they were able to work but who must confront real need for the first time in their old age may similarly be challenged or defeated by their dilemma.

Educational and intellectual differences. Among many elderly persons a low level of education is less a function of intellectual capacity than of educational opportunity. In earlier times, when the United States was principally rural, "book learning" was valued less than in today's urban society, because much of the preparation for effective living in a rural environment was acquired through experience rather than through books. A person who has thus spent only a·very few years in school may have become quite adept at living effectively or may have suffered greatly as a result of his or her limited education. Variations among the elderly in terms of formal education will greatly affect their individual perception of their problems and their ability to devise or accept a solution.

Gender differences. Most of today's elderly grew up and spent most of their lives in a world in which the roles of men and women differed sharply. They may, therefore, have more stereotypical thinking about men and women and their roles in society, and these stereotypes may be helpful or harmful. For example, a seemingly "dependent" woman who spent her days solving problems around the house while her husband was away at work may adapt more easily to the loss of her spouse than does an apparently more "independent" man who, after retiring from the job to which he devoted most of his daytime hours, suffers the death of his wife. She still has the familiar round of household tasks, duties, and chores, whereas he is left in an alien world, with no job, no fellow workers with whom to joke or chat, an unfamiliar home life of meals to cook and a household to care for, and no companion.

Differences in life experience. It cannot be stressed enough that the elderly are just you and I, grown older. We think of ourselves as unique, and so it is among the elderly, who have lived their lives not as members of an amorphous mass but, rather, as individuals. Among the elderly there are former explorers and opera singers, bridge builders and deepsea divers, bronco busters and violinists. Because many of the elderly will already have retired by the time they are seen by a service provider, it is easy to overlook the varied backgrounds they bring with them; however, the response of an elderly individual to the adversities, stresses, and problems of old age are largely conditioned by this person's earlier life experiences. In a more active phase of his or her life, did this person welcome change and obtain gratification from meeting challenges, or did he or she feel battered and beset by life when the inevitable problems of day-to-day living arose? An individual's response to problems is as diverse as, among other things, his or her life experiences.

Differences in health history. Increasingly, we are coming to appreciate the effects in old age of an individual's health history, whether this entails genetic components, such as a predisposition to certain disease conditions, or the influence of lifelong habits, such as diets high or low in fat, smoking versus nonsmoking, or a sedentary lifestyle versus one that is physically active. We are only now beginning to understand the full impact that early decisions in this regard make upon the well-being of the elderly.

Personality differences. Last, but by no means least, among the variables found between individuals, there is the fact of one's innate personality, over which an individual has little control. Although this is an elusive quality to quantify, its influence cannot be denied. Chown (1968) defined personality as "the gestalt (wholeness) of the individual's attitudes, emotions, motivations, and activity patterns—the impression a man [or woman] makes on others and the impression he [or she] makes on him[- or her]self." Personality is an adjustment pattern used by individuals to deal with internal and external demands imposed during the course of a lifetime. Unless research can effectively eliminate the possibility that such factors as income, marital status, trauma, sex, education, physical disability, social isolation, mobility, employment, and family might influence personality characteristics in later maturity, observed changes in social, emotional, and mental traits cannot be attributed to the aging process. What constitutes successful adjustment in later maturity is generally not defined in terms of specific behavioral patterns or activities. The degree of one's positive or negative adjustment rather than his or her overt behavior appears to constitute the most useful gauge of successful aging.

The human personality has secret springs of courage, along with the hidden fractures and flaws of potential frailties, and these, too, contribute to the differences found among all human beings, including the elderly.

AGING IS A PROCESS WITH MULTIPLE AREAS OF INVOLVEMENT

Aging is an extremely complex phenomenon. It involves changes in cellular structure, chemical activity, hormone production, behavior, cognitive functioning, sensory acuity, and personality. Social interactions, social roles, and social status change as a function of aging. Related to aging are modifications in patterns of work, leisure, and recreation. Therefore, problems among the elderly are often multidetermined—the result of a combination of interacting psychological, physical, social, and cultural forces.

Not only does aging take place along a number of different dimensions, but rates of aging along each dimension tend to vary from person to person. For example, we know that all people do not "look sixty-five" when they reach their sixty-fifth birthday and that all people do not maintain comparable levels of intellectual acuity at age eighty. Understanding and accepting the differential rates of aging between different people (regardless of age) is fundamental to our understanding of the aging process. In addition to the individual variations in life patterns, the elderly demonstrate great variability in level of functional impairment associated with the process of aging. Because of the multiplicity of factors involved in aging itself and in the problems faced by the aging individual, functioning, not chronology, must be the basis for geriatric assessment: age alone cannot be considered a reliable measure of an individual's physical changes, abilities, or limitations (Greene 1986).

Each human being is constantly aging in a number of ways, and different types of aging progress at different rates. If we study any one particular human being, we will inevitably notice that, for example, rate of social aging does not coincide precisely with rate of physical aging or that rate of functional aging may not have kept pace with psychological aging. The rapidity with which each type of aging occurs or progresses within the individual varies greatly.

There are three major categories of aging—biological, social, and psychological. There is constant interaction among the three categories, and change in any one dimension is likely to result in change in the others. Because of this interrelationship between categories, any changes, whether pronounced or subtle, must be considered and addressed by care providers.

Biological Changes

Age entails change. The biological changes of aging are inexorable and irreversible. They may be modified, retarded, accelerated, or ameliorated; aging itself, however, cannot be reversed. Although most changes associated with aging occur in a subtle manner and, indeed, are frequently imperceptible, some changes occur with relative rapidity and require an individual to adapt and adjust swiftly. Physical health impairments are among those changes that require the most far-reaching restructuring of one's life. One estimate is that five out of six people over age sixty-five have at least one chronic health problem (Harkins 1981).

Biological aging can precipitate change in the social and psychological areas. For example, as the number of brain cells decrease as a function of increased age (biological), changes may result in the ability to solve problems (psychological) or in the ability to engage in certain community activities (social). Even subtle deficits may exert profound effects. Consider, for example, the individual who has developed a slight hearing loss but is either unaware of that fact or chooses not to acknowledge it. He or she may become irritable over not understanding what is said or may not follow the thread of conversation in a group, making seemingly irrelevant comments, which might lead to erroneous conclusions that the individual is "a grouch" or "senile" and cause others to avoid him or her. This avoidance of social contact, in turn, can precipitate psychological difficulties—all because of a slight hearing deficit.

Social Changes

Retirement is an event that many people joyfully anticipate. Successful retirement, however, requires prior economic and social planning to enable the individual to fill the gaps that were once occupied by the tasks and social interactions of employment. When people retire without plans for leisure time, feelings of purposelessness and a lack of connection can develop (Osgood 1982). Once-longed-for privacy can turn into feelings of profound loneliness and isolation, as the hours once structured by employment and filled with interactions with coworkers loom long and frighteningly empty.

People who viewed retirement with eager anticipation all through their lives may discover that retirement brings an encompassing loss of self-identity and self-esteem, as they are forced to relinquish the roles that served to pattern their lives. The woman who built her life around her children and their activities might have, in another time, have made a smooth transition to devoting her time and attention to her grandchildren within the circle of the extended family.

156

Yet in today's mobile society children and grandchildren are likely to be far away, with only the occasional telephone call and hurried letters left to fill the gap. For such a woman, unaccustomed to building a social life outside the confines of her family, the hours can become long and empty.

A man who all his life has found his identity through his successful performance on his job may suddenly find himself, upon retiring, unable to get up in the morning, because nothing but empty hours stretch before him. The "psychological scaffold" provided by the workplace is gone, and the household chores or hobbies he thought would fill his time suddenly seem meaningless and unnecessary; soon he may also come to see himself and his life as devoid of meaning and unnecessary. People who have worked long hours throughout their lives in order to survive have had little need and little time to create a social network of their own and may feel totally at a loss about how to proceed, once the roles with which they have identified all their lives have come to an end.

For many elderly persons retirement also means a considerably diminished income, which in turn limits their social opportunities. A person who has barely enough money to pay the rent and/or make his or her house payment and put food on the table is not to be found on the cruises glowingly advertised to attract "senior citizens."

The result of all these factors is that many elderly individuals experience profound loneliness. Retirement, breakdown of the nuclear family, and the increasing development of age-segregated living communities have alienated the aged from many of their most meaningful group affiliations. "The all-too-limited outlets of religion, hobbies, television, pets, and a few acquaintances, which form the daily existence of so many of the elderly are not enough to satisfy emotional needs" (Butler and Lewis 1973). Indeed, the organizational regulations in many health care facilities, outlawing communal and conjugal living arrangements between elderly residents, actually serve to limit peer companionship and the emotional support elders might provide for one another (Albrecht and Adelman 1987).

Psychological Changes

All human beings suffer losses throughout the life cycle and must come to terms with them as best they can. Old age, however, combines two unfortunate sets of circumstances in this regard. First, losses in old age generally cover a broader spectrum, come in more rapid succession, and often are of a more serious nature. Second, the elderly person often must cope with these losses without adequate opportunity for substitution.

157

These multiple and cumulative losses can lead to depression, the most common mental health problem among the elderly (Zarit 1980). For example, the death of a spouse is an experience many older people must face; this entails not only the loss of a companion and/or household helper but may also mean loss of a source of income. It is understandable that such multiple losses, particularly in a vulnerable elderly person, can lead to profound depression. Untreated depression, in turn, can lead to numerous life-threatening problems, such as malnutrition, alcohol abuse, and attempted suicide as well as to a less dramatic but debilitating diminution in the quality of life of the elderly, through the day-to-day grayness of a life devoid of enthusiasm and joy.

AGING IS AN "UNEVEN" PROCESS

Added to the differences between individuals and the multiple factors that make up the aging process itself is the fact that people generally do not age "evenly," or in an overall manner. Most of us have had the experience of meeting and knowing an individual who "didn't look his or her age." Generally, what we mean is that the person was carefully groomed, had an interest in wearing up-to-date clothes, kept abreast of current events, and was an enthusiastic, interested, and interesting person. By the same token doctors' offices are filled with persons who are not so terribly old, chronologically, but who suffer multiple maladies, whether real or imagined, and who look and sound "old" to us.

There are many reasons for why a person seems old or young at any given chronological age, and the causes are as many and/or as complicated as the individual who is undergoing the aging. Chronic, debilitating diseases can make a person seem physically older than his or her chronological age. Isolation from society can cause a person to dress or groom him- or herself in a fashion that seems out of step with the current time and, therefore, makes the person look older. Lack of sufficient interpersonal interaction may leave visits to the doctor or to other health care providers as one of the few remaining ways in which the individual can secure much-needed attention and nurturance, causing elderly people to focus on minor or imagined illnesses and medications in an otherwise empty life. Finally, individuals may have been socialized to believe that one adopts, at some given chronological age, a way of behaving that has been designated as "appropriate" for the elderly. Often this mode of behavior is one that is inflicted and enforced by the younger generation, who find themselves embarrassed by their elderly relatives, should they insist on continuing to be thought of as, for example, sexually desirable men or women.

158

ASSESSING THE CLIENT

In order for older clients to receive care or services that are appropriate to their needs, caregivers must form an accurate assessment of the strengths and weaknesses of their clients. As we have seen, human problems, even those that appear to be simple, often involve a complex interplay of many factors. Rarely does the source of the client's problems reside solely within the individual or within his or her environment. Human beings are social creatures and are dependent upon other human beings and upon complex social institutions to meet their needs. Basic needs such as food, housing, clothing, and medical care require adequate economic means and the availability of goods and services. Educational, social, and recreational needs require interface with social institutions. Feeling close to and loved by others, having companionship, and experiencing a sense of longing require satisfactory social relationships within the family, within the individual's social network, and in the community.

Thus, an accurate assessment of the problems of a client system requires extensive knowledge about that system as well as consideration of the multiple systems that impinge upon it. Professionals, in assessing elderly clients, must be able to distinguish between age-related physical changes and underlying disease conditions. The assessment must take into account the client's reaction to his or her physical impairments and human losses and the effect on his or her self-esteem which changes in personal, occupational, social, and financial security may be producing.

The Initial Interview

Setting the atmosphere. The setting for the initial interview with a client should be as quiet and free from distracting interruptions as possible, and the client should be made to feel as comfortable as possible. Ideally, the interview should be conducted in a quiet, well-lighted room to offset the increased incidence of auditory and visual deficits among the elderly. Communication is enhanced if the professional sits in front of and at a slight angle to a client, a posture that demonstrates interest. Because high-frequency hearing is often diminished in elderly clients, speaking in a loud voice may lead to frustration for both the client and caregiver; rather, the interviewer should speak in clear, low tones.

The initial task is to establish rapport with the elderly client and any family members who are present. This is best accomplished by conducting the interview in a respectful and concerned manner. The professional should identify him- or herself to those present and, if necessary, clarify the purposes and goals of the visit at the beginning of the interview, rather than at a later time. It is especially important to address elderly clients by their surnames, unless they indicate that they prefer otherwise; casual use of first names may convey disrespect. To an individual whose self-esteem is already compromised, this seeming lack of respect from a younger person not known to the client may cause him or her to withdraw emotionally, destroying the potential bond of trust that must be established if the interaction is to be successful.

The professional should explain the purpose of routine procedures in clear, simple, and repetitive terms. The interview should be paced with the client's ability to communicate. It is essential that the caregiver remain flexible about the method in which the interview is conducted when reviewing the presenting problem. Older clients may attempt to avoid answering questions that highlight their physical, emotional, or social deficits by stating that they did not hear the question or commenting that the question is "silly" or undeserving of a response. This behavior may represent a healthy attempt at compensation; the care provider should not be deterred, however, and should press politely for specific responses to questions (Butler and Lewis 1973).

If conditions preclude obtaining accurate information firsthand, the family and other caregivers should be asked about the client's situation prior to the onset of the present problem. They may be able to provide essential historical information about the older client which otherwise would not be available. Yet the interviewer should be strongly warned against speaking primarily to the family member, referring to the client in the third person as if he or she were not present. This "self-defeating triangle" can be avoided by scheduling additional separate interviews with the client and with the family after outlining the general focus and goals of the examination in the initial interview. Privacy and self-determination of the client or patient must guide the assessment process (Cadieux et al. 1985).

The interviewer must be ever alert to any tone, comment, or action that could be interpreted by the elderly client as damaging to his or her self-esteem. As mentioned earlier, retirement from the work force frequently brings about abrupt changes in psychosocial status as a result of the loss of one's occupational productivity and accustomed roles in family interactions. The older person's perception of reduced respect from others owing to his or her decrease in income, goal-directed behaviors, and social activities may indeed be realistic, resulting in heightened sensitivity to anything that appears to threaten an already fragile sense of self-esteem. Sensitive discussion with a client about changes in living accommodations or the death of a spouse, as well as the loss of other family members or lifelong friends, may help the care provider identify the true onset of the client's present distress or circumstances.

Conducting the Initial Assessment

Every professional (e.g., physician, dentist, nurse, social worker, or lawyer) has a discipline-specific interview schedule and assessment format for his or her patients or clients. The evaluation performed by each professional may be so specific to his or her field, however, that not all aspects of the elderly client's circumstances are sufficiently investigated, and thus no overall profile emerges. Frequently, an elderly client must have contacts with numerous personnel and agencies in order to obtain needed health, social, or legal services. At each stop along the way an assessment must be carried out, whether through a formal questionnaire or a verbal interview.

The shortcoming of these multiple selective, discipline-specific interviews is that there is generally no single document existing which presents a balanced, overall view of the client and his or her situation. Attention has been paid, recently, to the overmedication of the elderly, when one physician is not informed of the medications being prescribed by another physician for the same patient. This same issue exists, in a broader sense, when there is no general, overall, broader profile of the elderly client. Such an "across-the-board" assessment should not be interpreted as a substitution for the discipline-oriented evaluations of such specialists as physicians or lawyers but, rather, as supplementary material, designed to augment and enhance the more specialized evaluation. Clearly, enhancing the health care or service provider's ability both to seek information effectively from an elderly client and to provide him or her with needed information will positively impact the interaction between the provider and the patient or client.

We believe a sensitive, caring, broad-spectrum initial geriatric assessment can benefit both the multiple concerned professionals who will ultimately be involved in providing care and services to the older client and the client him- or herself. This initial assessment can be documented in a "generic profile" form, which would be made part of the patient's or client's permanent record and would be updated with pertinent changes in status by subsequent interviewers. Details provided by such a generic profile tool can enable the practitioner to establish a dialogue with the client more quickly and can speed his or her decision making and problem solving. Additionally, the more general nature of such an assessment instrument may present aspects of the client's problems that would not normally be investigated by the particular professional being consulted but which may be valuable in the interaction taking place. The older client will, in

161

turn, be spared having to answer repeated questions about painful issues, such as the death of his or her spouse. Problem areas will be "flagged" for the professional, who can then concentrate on devising solutions more quickly and easily than if he or she had to cover the entire spectrum of questions all over again.

The geriatric assessment instrument must be one that can be administered easily, in the course of a normal intake interview, by any of the persons to whom the elderly client may appeal for initial assistance. First, the interviewing professional can observe and record his or her impressions about the client's general appearance, affect, intellect, and orientation, both before and during the interview. Throughout the interview simple, nonthreatening questions can be interjected which will enable the interviewer to assess the client's memory, judgment, and thought content. Careful attention to the client's responses and to the manner in which the responses are made will alert a care provider to the possibility of any underlying emotional disorder and the need for further interdisciplinary intervention (Cadieux et al. 1985).

AREAS TO BE COVERED

The following outline is intended to serve as a guide for the eight-step multidisciplinary assessment tool that we propose as an intake device for any professional first interviewing an older client. It can supplement whatever discipline-specific interview he or she may require for more detailed professional needs.

Appearance

Is the client neatly and appropriately dressed? Is his or her clothing clean? Is his or her hair neatly combed? Is the person clean? Poor self-care can be an indicator of the client's emotional state (e.g., depression), of inadequate housing arrangements, of economic distress, or of the individual's inability to care for him- or herself.

Does the client make eye contact when he or she interacts with the interviewer? What kind of posture, sitting or standing, does the client have? When asked a question, in what manner does the client respond? Does the client make any unusual movements or have any unusual movement patterns? A person who slumps in the chair, mumbling answers to the interviewer's questions and refusing to meet his or her eyes may be displaying the effects of depression, deep grief, or physical illness. Similarly, a person whose eyes dart unceasingly around the room, who fidgets relentlessly with his or her hair or clothing, and who answers questions not at all or only in fragments interspersed with long silences may be signaling the presence of emotional or physical problems that warrant further investigation.

Affect

The term *affect* refers to emotions or feelings. Most individuals experience periodic bouts with mood or emotional changes. They may feel blue, listless, or less hopeful than usual. The intensity, duration, and physical manifestations exhibited distinguish this behavior from normal depressive episodes.

It is understandable that a client may feel considerable stress, both from whatever underlying problems he or she is experiencing and from the interview situation itself. The interviewer, however, should be able to assess easily whether the general tenor of the client's mood and reactions is appropriate to the situation at hand. For a woman who has recently lost her husband, crying may represent an appropriate response, whereas weeping by an individual who can offer no reason for the tears may indicate underlying depression, a physical illness, or the presence of some life situation that is extremely upsetting to the client but which he or she does not feel free to discuss. Clearly, an individual who indicates grossly inappropriate affect, whatever the affect and whatever the situation, may be in need of further evaluation to determine the underlying cause.

Intellect

Intelligence is a hypothetical construct created by human beings in an attempt to explain individual differences. We assume its existence on the basis of observations that people exhibit different levels of abilities. This construct encompasses a multitude of specific and general abilities. For example, one's intellectual ability may be displayed in the form of verbal fluency, mechanical manipulation, spatial perception, abstract thinking, and information retention. Some people may be very talented in verbal communication but possess relatively little information retention. Findings have shown that many intellectual differences observed between various age groups cannot be attributed to growing old. Rather, such differences may reflect cohort or generational characteristics. Additionally, the data suggest that the normal aging process does not diminish an individual's ability to solve problems, to employ novel approaches, or to adopt an attitude of mental flexibility (Baltes et al. 1984). Certainly, the processes of mental aging are explained not only by normative data but by individual differences as well. As noted, older adults are a very diverse group.

The performance of individuals of similar educational backgrounds, regardless of age, tends to be more alike than the performance of individuals drawn randomly from the same age category. This correlation between educational level and intellectual performance may be attributable to initial similarities in aptitude as reflected by educational attainment.

The interviewer can ask, in a matter-of-fact manner, the last year of education attained by the client. It is not uncommon, among the elderly, for individuals to have had relatively little actual book learning. Nonetheless, they may have taught themselves occupations and skills, and gentle questioning should be able to establish a profile of the individual. Socioeconomic status can also be a determining factor. After acquiring a general idea of the individual's background, past accomplishments, and general intellectual level, careful inquiry about current knowledge can help give the interviewer some idea about the intellectual status of the client and help determine whether the individual is functioning at a level appropriate to his or her established capability.

Memory

There does seem to be some loss of memory ability as one reaches the later years, yet, again, there are individual differences. For most older people long-term memory (recalling distant events) tends to remain quite stable, and the ability to recount incidents that occurred decades before is not unusual. In later maturity declines in short-term memory are commonly noted (Baltes 1984).

Assessment of a client's short-term memory can be performed by asking several seemingly offhand questions, woven into the interview. "Did you have breakfast this morning? What did you eat?" Long-term memory can be similarly tested. "Do you remember where you lived the year you started school?" The interviewer must take care not to be too blatant with such questions, of course. An elderly client may become insulted and indignant if the questions or the manner of questioning are awkward or out of context. The skillful interviewer will manage such questions in a nonthreatening, conversational manner that implies interest in the client.

Judgment

If a client is engaging in behaviors that are clearly not beneficial to his or her well-being, does the client perceive the negative effect of these behaviors? Does the client even understand that a problem exists? If the client understands that a problem exists and that a solution must be sought, what solution does he or she propose? Does the client's suggestion demonstrate a sound grasp of the current situation and reflect logical problem-solving behavior? If the solutions to the problem at hand are all distasteful to the individual, is the person nonetheless able to recognize that one of the solutions must be implemented? For example, if an elderly person loses his or her spouse, is no longer able to care for him- or herself, and has no family support system, is this person able to recognize that a nursing home may be the only alternative?

Orientation

Orientation is an easily and accurately tested feature of elder assessment. Orientation about time (day, hour, year) is readily evaluated. Sense of place (where am I? what is this place?) and the ability to recognize familiar faces, in addition to oneself, should be included in the assessment of orientation.

Again, such questions should be incorporated into the interview in such a manner that a client does not realize he or she is being questioned in this regard. For example, recall of name and address can be confirmed through the simple device of asking the client for this information in order to fill out the basic intake form.

Level of Independence

Kastenbaum (1969) studied interdependent relationships among three adult generations drawn from the same families. Attention was given to assessing the cognitive and emotional aspects of dependency. Lack of knowledge of what to do and inadequate emotional support will affect the probability that individuals will fail to initiate activities that are in their own interests, thereby contributing to their dependency. The study indicated that the elders constituted the least-dependent generation in the study. They were much more affected, however, by the reduction in emotional support than were the other two generations. By maintaining strong affectional ties and mutually acceptable levels of association and reciprocity, the older generation can evaluate and balance their priorities (e.g., the need for emotional contact and the need to preserve independence and individuality).

Dependence or independence in elderly persons can be influenced by many factors of day-to-day life. Is the elderly person no longer able to afford to live independently and must therefore move in with a relative or friend? Do physical limitations make it impossible for the client to continue living in his or her accustomed home? Is the elderly individual someone who has been so dependent on a now deceased spouse that, now living alone, he or she is unable to assume the responsibility of increased independence? It is essential that the interviewer make an assessment of the client's degree of independence and attempt to determine the cause of whatever dependence the elderly person exhibits, if the professional is to be able to plan programs for the elderly individual. Sometimes elderly people are able and willing, perhaps even eager, to be far more independent than they are permitted to be by their grown children, and, in such cases, this fact must come to light, if the caregiver is to provide optimal solutions to the elder's problems.

Apparent Physical Limitations

As we have seen, physical limitations can profoundly influence the psychological and social well-being of the elderly individual; the impact of any physical impairment, therefore, is much more far-reaching than that of the particular physical limitation itself. The interviewer should observe the client carefully in order to note and record any seeming limitations. Is the individual's ability to move hampered in any way? Does sitting down or rising from a chair seem to cause the client pain? Is his or her handgrip strength sufficient for ordinary day-to-day activities? Is the client's sight sufficiently acute so that the client can still read normal newsprint, perhaps with the aid of glasses? If not, can the client read large-print magazines and books? Does the client have any apparent hearing loss? Often slight hearing loss may go unnoticed by the individual him- or herself but is sufficient to hamper interactions with other people. Because individuals often deny failing senses, both to themselves and to younger family members, sensitive feedback from the interviewer in these areas is essential; the client may be able to accept the objective, less personal observation of a stranger in this regard and allow him- or herself to be guided toward helpful programs, whereas such suggestions, coming from relatives, might be rejected.

ASSESSMENT AS AN ONGOING PROCESS

Assessment is an ongoing process from the moment of first contact with a client. During subsequent interviews practitioners weigh the significance of the client's behavior and any information revealed, including the thoughts, beliefs, and emotions expressed by the client. These moment-by-moment "mini-assessments" guide the care provider in deciding what aspects of the problem to explore at any given moment. A good client assessment contains a good general evaluation of all aspects of the elderly person, strengths and weaknesses, and becomes a living, growing portrait of the individual, as all relevant information gained in future exploration is incorporated into the picture.

To enhance the validity of this assessment it is valuable to involve clients in the process by sharing one's impressions with them about the nature of their problems and the possible solutions. By this process several goals may be accomplished simultaneously. First, by inviting the client's affirmation or disconfirmation of the professional's viewpoint or impression, the client, by virtue of having been invited to participate, is involved in the decision process. Second, by exposing his or her view of the situation and encouraging feedback, the professional may discover that the client views his or her problems within quite a different framework. It serves little for the professional to devise an elaborate solution, involving time, effort, and money, to a problem that the client views as insignificant. Third, the discussion serves to invite additional input and may reveal previously untapped strengths or identify other relevant resource systems that can be investigated or developed to remedy the client's difficulties. Only when the practitioner and the client reach an agreement about the nature of the problems involved are they ready to enter the process of negotiating, to set goals designed to alleviate the present conditions.

Crises for the aging can occur in multiple areas of an individual's life—physical health, role in the workplace or home, psychological well-being. Almost always the crisis of the original loss is multiplied manyfold by the vulnerability felt by the elderly, when they realize their lack of power—whether partial or complete, real or imagined—to compensate adequately for their losses. The ability of the caregiver to devise and facilitate solutions depends, therefore, not only on a complete and thorough analysis of the situation but also upon sensitive, empathetic communication with clients and their families, to understand how they view their own problems. The situations encountered are as varied as the individuals they affect. For example:

CASE EXAMPLE

Mildred and Jacob Green had been married for fifty-nine years. They were, as Mildred was fond of saying, like "two lovers who just look old." Both Mildred and Jacob had managed to remain healthy during the course of their marriage until recently, when Jacob, now eighty-three, suffered a severe stroke that left him paralyzed, incontinent, and barely able to speak. The geriatric nurse involved in coordinating a long-term care plan for Mr. Green must now determine the medical, social, financial, legal, and psychological needs of this client.

CASE EXAMPLE

Harry Bauer was, by almost anyone's standards, a happy and successful man. He was a highly paid executive in the company in which he had started as a mail room worker, thirty-eight years ago. He had a devoted wife and family, was physically in good health, financially secure, and a highly respected figure in the community. Suddenly, as he approached sixty, the chairman of the board of his firm gave him a harsh ultimatum: early retirement or transfer to an overseas position. Harry had postponed making retirement plans and was so overwrought by the disquieting confrontation in the chairman's office that he soon found himself seeking legal counseling.

CASE EXAMPLE

Tim and Barbara Harrington have reservations for a long-awaited dream vacation to Paris. The Harringtons go to visit his mother, Mabel, age eighty-five, who lives alone in a senior high-rise building. This is how the visit proceeds.

"Ma, we're leaving tomorrow. We'll be on vacation for two weeks. Don't forget: call cousin Buddy if you have problems."

"Why should I have problems!" Mabel retorts. "I live here alone all the time. I manage fine without you both, thank you."

"What's wrong, Ma? What did we do?" Tim is bewildered. Isn't Ma happy that he's realizing his dream vacation?

"Nothing. Nothing." His mother begins to sob. "Just go on about your business, and don't worry about me."

Tim and Barbara slink out of the apartment, chastened, guilty, low in spirits. Tim says, "I feel like a six-year-old who robbed the cookie jar. But I still don't know what's bugging her."

Barbara mutters between her teeth. "Well, she won again. Ruined our trip. And you'll be worrying every minute we're gone." This discussion brings Tim and Barbara to the office of a geropsychiatrist.

COMMUNICATION

The aim of the intervention process is to assist clients in reaching service goals. The best-designed, best-funded program in the world, however, is only as good as the communication established, one on one, between human beings: between the care provider and the client, the care provider and the family of the client, the care provider and his or her professional colleagues, and the care provider and the staff personnel of other agencies.

Care providers of the elderly in all the disciplines and elderly clients and their families depend upon communication to gather relevant information about social, legal, and health complaints, to elicit cooperation from others within the systems, as well as to provide relevant information to others within the systems. Health communication research has identified strong relationships between the quality of human dialogue in health care and the promotion of physical and psychological health, increases in health care provider and consumer satisfaction, and the accomplishment of health education (Mailbach and Kreps 1986).

Ultimately, the quality of services rendered by the entire social work and health care system—whether the intent be to provide elderly clients with social and emotional support; health, social, or legal evaluation feedback, or strategies to ameliorate adverse conditions—depends upon the ability of caregiving personnel to communicate in an effective, sensitive manner. This involves assessing clients' strengths and weaknesses, devising individualized plans to solve given problems, enlisting the input of clients and their families in regard to the problem and its prospective solution, and carrying out the intervention that will, it is hoped, benefit the client most.

The quality of interpersonal and organizational social work and health care communication with the aged can be enhanced by training care providers in both the role of communication and in the specific communication needs of the aged. These enhanced communication skills can increase a provider's ability to assess elderly clients effectively, to garner valuable and needed information, and to provide relevant information to other professionals in other agencies and disciplines on behalf of the elderly client.

To this end, enhanced communication, we propose a generic, noninvasive geriatric assessment instrument that will familiarize all service providers with the psychosocial status of their clients, based on the eight points previously mentioned. Such a generic assessment tool is not intended to supplant the discipline-specific interview and assessment schedules in use by the various health care and social and legal professionals. Rather, its purpose is to supplement such discipline-specific devices, by offering all service providers a kind of "thumbnail sketch" of the individual they find before them and of his or her situation and problems, thus enhancing service delivery by the entire service community encountered by the elderly client.

The multiple differences between elderly individuals, the complexity of the aging process itself, and the erratic, uneven manner in which people age make it extremely difficult for the care provider to identify the problems at hand, quantify their severity in any objective sense as well as in relation to the wishes of the client, and determine what solutions can be devised or whether solutions are possible or even necessary. Further, in the elderly, as in people of all ages, the presenting problem may not be the major or sole crisis. The client may be reluctant to reveal intimate matters or be fearful of appearing demanding or complaining. Clients may sometimes deny problems or even be unaware of them. A problem may not only have many causes; it may actually represent the combination of many problems. A skillful evaluator will search for possible combinations of problems, some of them perhaps less obvious than others but no less damaging. An assessment instrument such as the one we have proposed would guide the professional in attaining a balanced, overall viewpoint of each individual client and would provide, to other professionals, the benefits of this generic, overall profile—one not skewed by the particular disciplinary interest of the caregiver involved, by the nature of the problem being experienced, or by the way it is presented by the individual.

On the basis of such an assessment decisions can be made about reasonable, attainable, acceptable treatment goals: Can the problem at hand be reversed, or should the goal be merely to ameliorate it? If treatment is elected, should the goal be total recovery, partial restitution, maintaining the status quo, or, equally import, supporting the person during some inevitable decline? Is environmental change indicated? Does the individual need therapy, whether it be physical, social, or emotional? To answer these complex, interlocking questions it is necessary to assess the situation as accurately and clearly as possible, both to determine the nature of the problem and to quantify the resources available for its solution. It is necessary to know the older person's own emotional and physical capabilities, the assets available in his or her family and social structure, and the type of services and support available within the client's community.

Clearly, the length, style, and content of any assessment will depend upon the treatment method and setting under consideration as well as the individual's specific request for help. For example, an older person's request for assistance in dealing with the death of a spouse, placement in a nursing home, or information on a living will must necessarily require varying interview skills and evaluation schedules. Medical doctors, social service workers, mental health practitioners, lawyers, clergy, and all other professionals committed to working in behalf of older clients must collect information in a manner that ensures comprehensiveness without being rigid. Additionally, the method of obtaining the mass of data desired must be flexible in terms of how it is collected and who can collect it.

The data obtained should be recorded in a transferable form, capable of being passed from one professional to another and from one treatment setting to another, with the patient's or client's permission. The desirability of sharing such information among health providers is particularly important with older people, because numerous personnel may participate in their care, and the elderly frequently move from one setting or agency to another, as their conditions change. Sharing information saves time: it protects the client or patient from repeatedly having to answer the same questions; it records valuable information that may not be available later, should the client's or patient's mental or physical health deteriorate; and, as already mentioned, it offers a balanced overall view of the client or patient. Confidentiality can, of course, be maintained by sharing appropriately.

Careful, accurate evaluation is vital in any clinical situation, but, in gerontological health care and social work, assessment is especially critical. Persons initiating the request for help, either the older person or some interested third party, often ask questions that involve assessment. For example, concerned children, having decided that their father is suffering from symptoms of dementia, may ask, "Is my father getting senile?" Before initiating a treatment plan or involving other agencies or providers, the caregiver needs to evaluate and either confirm or fail to confirm the client's and/or family's formulation of the problem.

To summarize, some vital points must be noted in assessing older adults:

1. Although many older persons do not suffer from impairments stereotypically associated with age (e.g., sensory problems, cognitive impairment, or physical decrements), nor do these impairments necessarily occur in concert or at any given chronological age, it is vital that care providers be able to recognize these problems when they exist. The interviewer must be sensitive to such limitations as poor hearing, reduced vision, difficulty with speech, impaired mobility, and limited physical energy, both for the purposes of the interview and for the purpose of establishing a client's need for further care and services.

2. The interviewer must be sensitive to interpersonal differences among elderly clients, to include variations in formal education and verbal skills, cultural and ethnic differences in communication styles, variations in socialization, and multiple attitudes, beliefs, and interests. The aged, as a group, currently have less formal education than the general population; as a result, some older persons may not possess the verbal skills necessary to communicate complex feeling states. It is essential that care providers learn to communicate clearly, avoiding professional jargon and presenting concepts and methods in a concrete, straightforward fashion.

3. Due to the difference in age between elderly clients and most caregivers, clients may feel that interviewers cannot possibly understand them and their problems. Care providers must be prepared to address, in a nondefensive way, such questions as, "How can you understand or help me? You're so young." They must be able to assure their clients that their clinical or social work expertise is based on knowledge, training, and self-awareness, rather than age. If the inter-

171

view is conducted with sensitivity, not only to the client's problems but also to the fact that the client is a human being, age will cease to be an issue. The interviewer must never forget that the client did not ask to be old, that the client is suffering very real losses, and that, although the dilemma may often defy solution, it is one that is universal and deserving of empathy, kindness, and, above all, respect for the struggles and pain of another human being.

4. Once having been obtained, the data from such a broad-based, overall evaluation should be recorded and made part of the patient's or client's permanent file, so that other professionals interviewing that person at a later date will have the benefit of the initial "generic" assessment to serve as a baseline for their own observations. This baseline generic profile will help provide them with an overall picture of the patient or client and will serve as a basis of comparison for gauging the later status of the client or patient.

Quality services and care for older adults are a hallmark of a humane society. Older adults have lived their lives in service to that society and deserve society's best efforts in their latter years to enable them to complete their lives in comfort and dignity. They are not a homogeneous group of people suffering a homogeneous cluster of ills and failings; they are all of us grown older. Careful evaluation of this complex group of people and their multiple problems is essential if existing services are to be able to stretch to encompass this burgeoning age group. Careful initial assessment, employing an instrument that will record the examiner's observations and comments concerning a broad-spectrum, overall view of the client, is the first step toward diagnosing and investigating the patient's or client's concerns and problems. Making this initial generic evaluation available to assist future caregivers in their own, more specialized evaluations is a valuable second step toward providing, for our elders, the high-quality, personalized care they so richly deserve.

REFERENCES

Albrecht, T., and M. Adelman. (1987). *Communicating social support.* Newbury Park, Calif.: Sage.

Baltes, P. B., and O. G. Brim Jr., eds. (1984). *Life-span development and behavior,* vol. 6. Orlando, Fla.: Academic Press.

Butler, R., and M. Lewis. (1973). *Aging and mental health.* St. Louis: C. V. Mosby.

Cadieux, R. J., J. D. Kales, and L. Zimmerman. (1985). Comprehensive assessment of the elderly patient. *American Family Physician* 31, no. 5: 105–11.

Chown, S. M. (1968). Personality and aging. In *Theory and methods of research on aging,* ed. K. W. Schaie, 134–57. Morgantown: West Virginia University Press.

Dana, Bess, and Cecil Sheps. (1973). Trends and issues in interprofessional education: Pride, prejudice, and progress. In Elements of social work practice, by Delwin Anderson. Paper presented at the Annual Meeting and Workshop, Society for Hospital Social Work Directors, Denver, 22 September.

Greene, R. R. (1986). *Social work with the aged and their families.* New York: Aldine De Gruyter.

Harkins, E. B. (1981). *Social and health factors in long-term care: Findings from the statewide survey of older Virginians.* Richmond: Virginia Commonwealth University, Virginia Center on Aging.

Kastenbaum, R. (1969). *The dependencies of old people.* University of Michigan. Monograph.

Mailbach, E. W., and G. L. Kreps. (1986). Communicating with patients: Primary care physicians' perspectives on cancer prevention, screening, and education. Paper presented to the International Conference on Doctor-Patient Communication, Center for Studies in Family Medicine, University of Western Ontario, London, Ont.

Osgood, N. (1982). *Life after work: Retirement, leisure, recreation and the elderly.* New York: Praeger.

Shulman, B., and R. Berman. (1988). *How to survive your aging parents.* Chicago: Surrey Books.

Zarit, S. H. (1980). *Aging and mental disorders.* New York: Macmillan.

Chapter 11

THE COORDINATION OF A REFERRAL AND TREATMENT PLAN

Role clarity and cooperation are the necessary prerequisites for the implementation of a multidisciplinary approach for serving older adults in the community. The preceding two chapters defined the professional roles of the various elder practitioners and the areas to be included in a generic elder assessment. The present chapter focuses on the establishment of a collaborative multidisciplinary approach to service. The present chapter focuses on what collaboration is, how collaborative networks are established, and what mechanisms exist for fostering collaboration and overcoming obstacles to collaboration.

COLLABORATION

The importance of effective collaboration is not a nascent concern. Mullaney, Fox, and Liston (1974) have addressed the problem of improving relations between the nursing and social work professions, by emphasizing the need for better understanding among professions to accomplish more effective collaboration. Dana (1973) advised that interprofessional behavior requires "knowledge, values and skills that transcend the professions" and the acknowledgment of "limitations as well as the possibilities within one's own professional armamentarium." In more recent years the professional literature has concentrated on the need for more coordinated discharge planning (Foster and Brown 1978; Shulman and Tuzman 1980). Continued interest in transprofessional activity derives from the understanding that multiprofessional relationships have important implications for the cost-effectiveness of service delivery. For example, better coordination of outside services can avert the need for costly hospitalizations. Total quality management (TQM) is a contemporary management strategy that emphasizes the impact of coordination upon overall efficiency and quality in service delivery. TQM represents a comprehensive application of the principles of system coordination. The focus of scholarship, however, has remained the formal organization and ensuring the access of the elderly client to formal outside services. The interaction of the various independent professionals in the life of the community elderly virtually has been ignored.

CONCEPTS DERIVED FROM ROLE THEORY

Role theory provides a useful organizing framework for an analysis of collaboration. Collaboration is a specific type of multidisciplinary or interprofessional approach which represents the standard being promoted in this book.

Role theory defines human organizations and institutions as systems of roles (Katz and Kahn 1978). A role constitutes activities one would expect to perform as an occupant of a given status or position. Role theory acknowledges that organizations are based on a particular set of norms and values, in addition to roles. Norms are standardized requirements of behavior in a system and include role requirements. Norms range from internal agency policies to state regulations and statutes. At present the interprofessional activities of independent practitioners are not highly regulated. Regulations governing home care and discharge planning have some implications for professional liability in ensuring patient safety; however, interprofessional role connections are not neatly spelled out in any legislation. Most independent practitioners do not follow any strict guidelines for collaborating with professionals from other disciplines. Norms and values provide reinforcement for role requirements.

Roles are the most concrete behavioral sanction in that they simply define what you do, rather than what you must or should, do (Katz and Kahn 1978). The role relationship represents the nature of the interaction between different role performers (Nathanson 1984). The role relationship for collaboration represents a role performer's interaction with other professionals toward a specific type of cooperative effort.

THE MULTIDISCIPLINARY MODEL

The Coordination of a Referral and Treatment Plan

The multidisciplinary model deliberately places each role performer at the beginning of the referral exchange process. No single role performer is viewed as the general anchor in the scheme, which represents a departure from more traditional referral processes; organizationally based collaborative models of interaction tend to place the social worker or nurse at the center of the collaborative exchange process. In the present scheme the primary professional in the client's or patient's experience is the natural anchor in the referral process (see fig. 7). Since there are no formal constraints on the various disciplines included in the collaborative effort, it is ethically incumbent upon each role performer to initiate appropriate referrals. This serves to protect individuals from the pitfalls of a fragmented delivery system.

IMPLEMENTATION OF THE MODEL

Having identified the various professional roles involved (see chap. 8) and the nature of the role relationship for collaboration, it is necessary to examine the issue of how an independent practitioner begins to build a collaborative multidisciplinary network. Unlike an organization bounded by walls, the community service field is a wide-open system. There are no internal agency policies to govern interdisciplinary activities. There are few regulatory limits. In

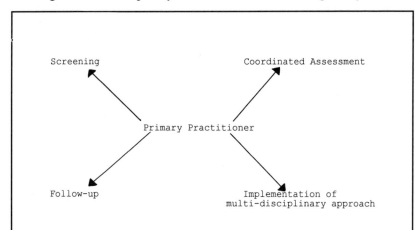

Screening   Coordinated Assessment

Primary Practitioner

Follow-up   Implementation of multi-disciplinary approach

FIG. 7. THE COORDINATION OF A REFERRAL AND TREATMENT PLAN

This figure illustrates the circularity of the patient's or client's movement through the system. The primary practitioner serves as the fulcrum around which the individual moves.

fact, negligence and malpractice law has more influence than any formal statute in constraining the referral practices of community-based professionals. The question of how to build an interdisciplinary network has no single answer. Each practitioner networks in his or her own way. There are, however, certain principles that can be employed in ensuring effective coordination.

Know the scope and limits of one's responsibility. The importance of clarifying one's own tasks and the limitations of one's professional activities cannot be overstated. Professional associations provide sanctions for their members' professional roles. Public health statutes and negligence and contract law protect the service recipient, to a certain extent, from capricious and incompetent practices. Yet, as pointed out in chapter 9, there is a potential for overlap in defining the tasks of the various professions. The independent practitioner has to be clear about what he or she considers the stated professional purpose. The social worker, for example, has to decide whether case management or psychotherapy, or both, describe the scope of professional responsibility. The psychiatrist has to decide whether to include psychotherapy within the scope of his or her responsibilities or to concentrate exclusively on biopsychiatric treatment. The lawyer has to determine whether he or she plans to serve as financial advisor or to restrict his or her practice to specific areas of the law, such as application for benefits or planning for incapacity. A clear understanding of one's own tasks prepares the way for more effective coordination with other professionals who are involved.

Access other disciplines. How does one go about establishing working relationships with other private practitioners or community agencies? The key to forming effective referral networks is getting to know other practitioners or agencies in one's catchment area. This is, of course, more difficult in large metropolitan areas than in small towns. In large cities, however, one has the advantage of choice. Professional meetings and conferences provide a direct mechanism for establishing connections. State gerontological society conferences, for example, provide an excellent opportunity for interdisciplinary networking. Professional associations, such as the local bar association, will provide the names of individuals specializing in elder law in the local community. Some communities have interagency aging councils or health task forces that can be accessed through the local area office for aging (AAA) or health systems agency (HSA). These can serve as sources for referral, as can recommendations by other practitioners. There is no cut-and-dried methodology for establishing contacts.

Yet relationships of trust do not happen by chance. The establishment of a role relationship with another professional results from the mutual appreciation

177

and support of each other's service objectives. In other words, after clarifying one's own role, one must understand the other's role and the nature of the role relationship. A typical question that might be addressed is: Under what circumstances would it be appropriate to refer a client or patient? Relationships of trust can only be built over time and experience with each other's practice habits. A period of testing is to be expected, and it may be found that certain individuals are inappropriate as sources of continuous consultation.

One of the documented problems with certain pre-paid group practices is that referrals for consultation are arbitrary and that quality suffers when physicians, for example, do not have discretion in their choice of consultants. Discretion in the area of referrals is one way in which the medical profession has maintained accountability within its ranks; in other words, a doctor who is viewed as incapable or substandard does not receive referrals. Experience has taught that discretion in choice of consultants serves as a useful informal constraint upon professional behavior. Yet, to realize the full potential of this liberty, professionals must discriminate as effectively in making interdisciplinary connections as in making intradisciplinary connections. This involves understanding the nature of the other's role as well as one's own.

Maintain consistent contact with other professionals. Once one has completed the task of establishing linkages with other professionals in the community, the elder practitioner must be prepared to follow up on referrals. Medical doctors, who are accustomed to working autonomously, may be more comfortable delegating the responsibility for follow-up to a staff member, such as a social worker, geriatric case manager, or nurse. A psychologist who restricts the scope of responsibility to treatment and does not view resource coordination as part of the professional role can utilize the services of a geriatric case manager to coordinate and follow up on a patient's continuity of care requirements. The authors endorse a situational approach to implementing a collaborative model of community service. The authors respect the fact that the collaborative role relationship may not be as compatible with the practices of certain professions as it is with those of others. There is no single solution to working out the methods by which the community practitioner coordinates his or her activities with other practitioners. The critical factor is that a method is worked out.

FOSTERING COLLABORATION

There are two directions to go in fostering collaboration. The first is really more a matter of forcing, rather than fostering. Collaboration can, and may, be legislated. This has already happened to a large degree in hospital discharge planning. The statutes and regulations affecting hospital discharge planning or continuity of care management are promulgated by a variety of federal, state, and local legislative bodies and agencies, including state health departments, the Joint Commission on Accreditation of Health Organizations (JCAHO), and the Professional Review Organization (PRO), which is the current federal program for utilization review of Medicare beneficiaries. In addition, the Health Care Financing Administration (HCFA) has instituted fee restrictions for outpatient services provided by professionals participating in the Medicare program, thereby exercising the proverbial "power of the purse strings" approach to regulation.

More regulation seems to be on the horizon with the development of new federal health care legislative packages. Pre-paid group practices or managed-care operations are expected to become more central to health care delivery. The implications of these trends for a model of multidisciplinary community practice are discussed in the next chapter. For present purposes, suffice it to say that more rules can be expected. If independent community practice is to survive, and if professionals are to maintain their present levels of discretion in treatment decisions, then they have to take responsibility for developing and enforcing professional standards for interdisciplinary as well as intradisciplinary behavior. This book represents a beginning step toward the goal of promoting interprofessional accountability and avoiding unnecessary governmental interference.

This brings us to the second means for fostering collaboration. It concerns the willingness by professionals to collaborate. This willingness derives from a preference for this type of role relationship. A willingness to collaborate develops when there is perceived value in collaborating. Why would a professional want to collaborate? The answer to that question is, "It depends." Many professionals will be motivated by the objective of providing a comprehensive service. Others may be motivated by less worthy objectives, for example, to avoid the risk of a negligence action or to increase their referral bases. Most are motivated by some combination of financial and quality objectives. The independent professional can seek to reinforce a willingness to cooperate in others, by identifying the nature of the reciprocity that grows out of such a group effort. The benefits of the mutual exchange can and should unabashedly be highlighted.

Values provide an internal motivation or control for behavior, whereas norms and rules represent external constraints. The *locus of control theory* offers an explanation of the relative influence of the different types of controls. In other words, locus of control theory seeks to explain whether individuals are more influenced more by internal motivations or, rather, by outside pressures. Although locus of control theory suggests that intrinsic incentives are sufficient

179

for increasing motivation among certain individuals, there will be an additional mix of intrinsic motivations and extrinsic incentives when the extrinsic incentive does not challenge a person's experience of him- or herself as self-determining (Gold 1990). Thus, professional norms or rules of conduct which develop from a value base provide the strongest combined incentive for motivating certain behaviors.

SPECIFIC STRATEGIES FOR IMPLEMENTING THE COLLABORATIVE MODEL

There are specific strategies that have proven effective in promoting collaboration. What follows is a delineation of these strategies:

1. Establish a consensus with other professionals regarding the purpose of the collaboration. Just as a contract is effective in clarifying and outlining the goals of one's professional interchange with a client or patient, a contract can be effective in establishing the terms of the relationship with other practitioners. "What are we doing together?" is the question that must be addressed. Careful attention to this aspect of practice can avoid confusion for clients as well as colleagues.

2. Define the nature of each other's professional tasks. If there is an overlap in the job description of a social worker and a psychiatrist, for example, it is necessary to establish a point of agreement regarding the scope and limits of each other's work with mutual patients.

3. Establish an agreement regarding preferred outcomes for elderly clients or patients. Does the attorney share the same objectives for the client as the geriatric case manager? For example, the principle of the least restrictive alternative must be balanced against the client's need for protection in planning for incapacity. The attorney and the geriatric case manager ought to be able to come to some agreement regarding preferred outcomes in specific situations.

The organizing principle behind these strategies is that of collaboration based on consensus. This must address the reason for working together, the ways of working, and the objectives of the work.

OBSTACLES TO COLLABORATION

The path to collaboration can be expected to have a few rough spots. There are several predictable problems that may arise at different stages of the process, including the following.

1. Failure to establish consensus regarding the reason for the collaboration, the styles of working together, and the objectives. An interdisciplinary connection will most certainly fail to produce positive results if the professionals involved do not agree on the purpose and mode of collaborating. For example, attorneys are client advocates; physicians tend to align themselves with hospital discharge policy; social workers tend to find themselves in the often unenviable position of trying to mediate the demands of a health care system and the rights of an individual. How can all of these people cooperate in promoting the best interest of the clients they serve, when the definition of the client varies from one professional to the other? This question is not easily answered. In the authors' experience establishing the right match is crucial in forming a collaborative relationship. One should at least be able to agree with those professionals one chooses as colleagues. When a physician encounters a legal problem with an office patient, the physician is less constrained by conflicting organizational demands than if the patient were a hospital inpatient. This places community practitioners at an advantage over institutional employees in being able to respond to the needs of the client without organizational encumbrance. The price of discretion, however, is greater accountability to act in the client's best interest. This trust is not to be taken lightly.

2. Territoriality. Professionals in private practice are entrepreneurial. It is no use denying this fact. Consequently, suspicion may surround the involvement of other professionals in one's practice. Clear guidelines for referral and intervention can ease tensions among professionals. Additionally, collaboration with other professionals has the advantage of liberating practitioners to do what they have been trained to do; for example, if an attorney can rely on a social worker or psychologist to mediate family tensions, the attorney is freer to concentrate on legal concerns. The cost-effectiveness of appropriate delegation of responsibility is evidenced in cost savings for families and increased confidence among service providers.

3. Family dynamics. Never to be underestimated is the importance of the family in matters pertaining to continuity of care planning for an aging relative. Although this model places the older client or patient in the center of the professional's sphere of concern, the family can never be disregarded. Families can create conflicts. Difficulties over settlement of an estate often emanate from family disputes over the distribution of funds, and family conflicts over long-term care planning for

181

an elderly individual are commonplace. Family conflicts can be minimized, however, by involving family members in the planning from the start, if the older individual is willing to have them participate in the process. It is important to consider that older people are particularly vulnerable to the influence of family members because of their increased fears of dependency. Therefore, primary professionals involved with the older person must guard against the potential for family coercion by advocating, when necessary, on behalf of the older person. Families can also be great sources of assistance in continuity of care planning. Daughters are the primary caregivers for their mothers. Therefore, it is important that respect for the caregiver's role be carefully balanced against concern for the older individual's autonomy in health care decision making.

4. Crisis situations. Crises, it is hoped, can be avoided with careful planning. Until people become more accustomed to seeking professional help before a problem develops, however, professionals are going to continue to be besieged by families in crisis. "I must get my mother into a nursing home tomorrow"; "My father is no longer able to manage his finances"; "Ever since my mother suffered a fall six months ago, she has been sullen and has been eating poorly"—appeals for help such as these are not unusual in elder practice.

Sometimes crises arise because of upsets in the delivery of professional services or problems in the coordination of services. For example, the trusted home health aide must resign; the patient is getting physically stronger but is not motivated to get out of bed; or the cost of home health services has resulted in the older person's near impoverishment. Careful screening of needs and preventive intervention can help to avert some of these problems or at least avoid further difficulty. The effective handling of the situation will fall to the primary professional, whose best defense in a crisis is his or her interdisciplinary network. The network is not only useful in reducing stress for the client but is also a useful resource for professionals in reducing obstacles to the completion of their tasks.

APPLICATION OF THE MODEL

The case vignette that follows illustrates the implementation of a collaborative approach in multidisciplinary elder practice and some of its common pitfalls.

CASE EXAMPLE

Rose L. is a ninety-one-year-old white woman who has been widowed for the last ten years. Her husband left her with relative financial security, yet she has been drawing upon the principal in order to meet her monthly expenses. She has one hundred thousand dollars remaining in her estate and has been drawing approximately ten thousand dollars per year from the total to supplement her income from social security. Rose L. is concerned about her ability to maintain her personal and financial independence in light of her increasing physical frailty. Although her health generally is good, she suffers from a degenerative arthritic condition, which makes it difficult for her to ambulate and to complete household chores such as shopping, cleaning, and cooking.

Rose L. has no children, but has a variety of nieces and nephews who live in different parts of the country from her. Two of these individuals, a niece and a nephew, help to coordinate the resources required for her continuity of care. Rose L. has an attorney, who oversees her financial affairs. For example, the attorney monitors the reasonableness of her expenditures and files her income taxes. Rose L.'s nephew has durable power of attorney.

Rose L. is considering the possibility of moving to a home for adults, where she can receive supportive services. She has not been sleeping well and has been in daily phone contact with her attorney. The attorney has referred Rose L. to a geriatric case manager to assess her service needs and to assist with resource coordination. The geriatric case manager and Rose L. agree to investigate living alternatives. Meanwhile, Rose L. continues to have difficulty sleeping and, ultimately, discloses to the case manager her reservations about leaving her home. The geriatric case manager arranges for part-time home care as an alternative to institutional placement. This plan works for a while, until Rose L.'s personal care needs begin to escalate. It is apparent that she needs at least eight hours of home care per day. The home care worker's hours are increased. The cost of the home care is approximately one hundred dollars a day.

The family would like Rose L. to reconsider institutional placement. After deliberation with the family Rose L. goes along with this plan. Rose L. asks the geriatric case manager to renew the search for an appropriate nursing home. The attorney is told of this turn of events and goes to talk with Rose L. Rose L. admits that she is not pleased with the plan, and the attorney in turn discusses her reluctance with her niece and nephew. The niece and nephew argue that nursing home placement is best for Rose L. under the circumstances, and Rose L., apathetically, supports their position. Plans are made for placement.

This scenario represents the expedient implementation of a plan for the continuing care of a client. Some of the issues that are raised regard the lack of clear role responsibilities; the failure to address the client's depression; the neglect of the client's true wishes; the lack of clear consensus regarding the geriatric case manager's objectives for the client and those of the attorney; the lack of inclusion of other key human service professionals in the planning, for example, the geriatrician or the geropsychotherapist; and the smoothing over of conflicts. Careful attention to the following questions may have helped to avert some of the problems encountered in implementing a care program for Rose L.

1. How can one ensure a comprehensive screening of the client's needs?

2. Which professional should conduct the screening?

3. What could the two professionals have done to better coordinate their own roles?

4. What could the attorney and geriatric case manager have done to better coordinate their roles with that of the family?

5. What options could have been presented for the client's continued care?

6. What are the pros and cons of the various options?

7. How might other professionals have been engaged to ensure comprehensive care for the client?

8. How might the disagreement over placement have been addressed to the advantage of both the client and her family?

9. Do the professionals agree on who is the primary client?

10. How could a consensus between the professionals regarding the preferred outcome for the client have helped to guide their respective activities?

These questions help focus the professionals' attention on the purpose and process of their teamwork. The model being presented requires that as much consideration be given to the nature of the collaboration as to the independent task requirements of the various role performers. A key principle of this approach is not to ignore conflicts among role performers, including the client and the family, but, rather, to identify points of compromise, if possible, among the various role performers. The Multidisciplinary Screening Instrument (MSI) is a tool used to foster comprehensive assessment and to provide for comprehensive care.

Professionals may view their goals for their clients or patients differently. Attorneys, for example, tend to see themselves as patient advocates, which could tend to foster an adversarial climate for an exchange with other professionals or family members. Professionals have to come to some agreement regarding role responsibilities and preferred outcomes for clients or patients. This type of negotiation requires that each be willing to identify the points of compromise among their separate professional agendas. This mediation of needs and goals may be the hardest step to accomplish in the multidisciplinary approach.

A lack of clarity in objectives, however, either will result in a sidestepping of issues or overwhelming tension, resistance, and confusion. Sometimes people may not agree about value issues but are able to agree on an operational level. It is no use arguing the right to the least restrictive alternative in continuity of care planning with a family member or professional caregiver who does not share the same view. There may, however, be room for agreement among different perspectives when the practical consequences of a particular treatment or caregiving option are spelled out. For example, forcing an older person to go to a nursing home when it can be avoided can result in adverse consequences to the person's mental and physical health. A paternalistic physician may be able to let go of his or her need to protect the older person from the risks involved in independent living if the potential negative consequences of placement are highlighted. Conversely, the overzealous attorney who firmly supports the client's right to make his or her own decisions may be moved by the reality of an ailing caregiver's own tribulations in struggling to cope with balancing responsibilities and personal needs. The law defines a variety of human rights and protective interventions, but there are many gray areas. It is up to the professionals involved to see that plans are not made for the sake of expediency or in order to support a certain biased position. They should be made in the interest of the client, according to that person's perception of his or her own welfare, and in the interest of the principal caregivers, according to their perceived needs. When there is a conflict, the professionals must be prepared to mediate it quickly, thus showing their concern and commitment to all of the principals involved.

This chapter provides a theoretical framework for implementing a multidisciplinary approach to serving the elderly in the community. Role theory provides the organizing framework for identifying the tasks of the various human service providers and for describing the nature of the role relationships among them. The approach calls for clarity and cooperation in carrying out interdisciplinary activities and cautions against certain common obstacles to cooperation or clarification. These obstacles include problems in contracting or achieving consensus regarding the goals for the particular collaborative effort as well as failures in providing a comprehensive assessment of the client's needs and effectively responding to these needs. The multidisciplinary model employs a mediating approach to resolve disputes among role performers. The key to successful mediation is viewed as the ability to identify the quid pro quo, or the opportunities for reciprocity among the client, family members, and professionals.

REFERENCES

Dana, B., and C. Sheps. (1973). Trends and issues in interprofessional education: Pride, prejudice and progress. In Elements of social work practice, by Delwin Anderson. Paper presented at the Annual Meeting and Workshop, Society for Hospital Social Work Directors, Denver, 22 September.

Foster, Z., and D. Brown. (1987). The social work role in hospital discharge planning. *Social Work in Health Care* 4, no. 1 (Fall): 55–63.

Gold, N. (1990). Motivation: The crucial but unexplored component of social work practice. *Social Work* 35, no. 1 (January): 49–56.

Katz, D., and R. Kahn. (1978). *The social psychology of organizations.* New York: John Wiley and Sons.

Mullaney, J., R. Fox, and M. Liston. (1974). Clinical nurse specialist and social work—clarifying the roles. *Nursing Outlook* 22, no. 11: 712–18.

Nathanson, I. (1984). Patterns of adaptation of social workers to the acute care setting. Ph.D. diss., Yeshiva University.

Shulman, L., and L. Tuzman. (1980). Discharge planning—social work perspective. *Quarterly Review Bulletin* (October): 3–7.

Chapter 12

IMPLICATIONS OF
THE MULTIDISCIPLINARY APPROACH

This chapter explores the implications of a multidisciplinary approach to service delivery, education and training, and research and policy development. The authors also examine some of the obstacles that may need to be overcome in promoting a multidisciplinary approach.

IMPLICATIONS FOR SERVICE DELIVERY

The importance of the multidisciplinary approach is inherent in its potential impact upon the provision of services to the elderly in the community. The multidisciplinary approach outlined in this book is designed to reshape the nature of professional practice by providing a blueprint for the integration of professional services. The beauty of this approach is its relative simplicity. While policy makers are attempting to find effective solutions to gaps in the delivery of human services, many of which would require radical shifts in the organization of the delivery of health and human services, this approach recognizes the potential for grassroots reorganization that can take place within the constraints of any broad-scale institutional framework. In other words, this model is applicable whether community health care is arranged according to principles of pre-paid group health organizations, which emphasize utilization review and prevention, or it continues to be arranged according to traditional standards of fee-for-service solo practice, which emphasize consumer choice and medical expertise in health care decision making.

The collaborative techniques advanced in this book can be incorporated into practice now and always. They are, for all intents and purposes, basic. They are such a fundamental part of good practice that they can easily be overlooked as being negligible additions to the professional armamentarium. And yet comprehensive assessment and collaboration are as critically basic to a professional's skillfulness as medical diagnosis is to a physician or taking a deposition is to a trial attorney. Moreover, interdisciplinary behavior impacts the total system of organization, while the private relationship between an independent practitioner and his or her client or patient does not, however positive the outcome of the helping relationship.

Charlie Chaplin memorialized the sense of detachment and lack of gratification associated with working on an assembly line and performing only part of a job in the silent film classic *Modern Times*. Professionals like to think of themselves as performing and expecting others to perform their work according to a professional whole-task system. With increased specialization and bureaucratic constraints most professionals are frustrated by what are viewed as encroachments upon their autonomy. Perhaps the single most important implication for service delivery of this approach regards professional autonomy. A multidisciplinary approach to service delivery can offset a lack of fulfillment by providing professionals with a sense of continuity and task completion.

Professions are distinguished by a number of features, including their expertise and authority. The professions are distinguished from one another on the basis of variations in service mission and professional function. Paradoxically, increased collaboration, while creating greater fluidity among professionals, would serve to hone professional edges, by encouraging clarification about one's professional function.

With more and more emphasis being placed on cost containment, professions must establish new institutional grounds for legitimacy. Even medical doctors are no longer revered simply on the basis of their traditional status in the medical hierarchy. Professions have to reexamine their underpinnings and elaborate their objectives in our new consumer-oriented service arena. The public wants to know what it is getting. The model described in these pages is developed from a conception of the needs of the older service recipient. As consumers become more educated, they will demand more for their money. It is a matter of common sense that those professionals who anticipate the needs of their clients will have an edge in the service marketplace. Similarly, those professions that encourage collaboration as a standard of conduct will better ensure public regard for their authority and autonomy. In defining their limits, they will, in fact, be defining their powers.

IMPLICATIONS FOR EDUCATION AND TRAINING

What better place to advance principles of practice than in our professional schools and training institutions? The implications for education and training of a multidisciplinary approach to serving the elderly are as profound as the influence of education is to the socialization of professionals to their roles. Professionals are trained to perform their roles according to the values and techniques that describe ethical and competent practice. The multidisciplinary approach derives from a conception of what is right as well as what is technically effective in delivering community services to the elderly. The education of professionals must incorporate a consideration of both the ethical and technical applications of a collaborative approach. It is not enough to pay lip service to the merits of collaboration and to suggest that professionals cooperate with one another in providing a comprehensive service. Each profession has the responsibility of detailing the specific implications of collaboration for its practitioners and of teaching students the methods of collaboration. Just as most professional degree programs include courses in administrative responsibility or ethics, professional syllabi should include a focus on developing multidisciplinary connections.

It is the responsibility of voluntary accrediting bodies to promulgate standards for educational curricula. State licensing agencies also mandate requirements for professional practice. Rather than wait for the government to regulate interdisciplinary activities, professional accrediting bodies would do well to promote their own standards for multidisciplinary practice.

The techniques outlined in this book provide a basic outline of the various dimensions of a multidisciplinary approach. The book can serve as the nucleus of an educational program for students in the various disciplines.

IMPLICATIONS FOR RESEARCH

Many questions will arise regarding the cost-effectiveness of a multidisciplinary approach. These types of questions open the door to investigations of such issues as time saving, cost saving, and the quality of care. Scientific research is very valuable in elucidating the advantages and disadvantages of specific organizational schemes. Is it more cost-effective for an attorney to work with a geriatric case manager than to assume the responsibility for coordinating resources? Are health maintenance organizations more conducive to promoting multidisciplinary cooperation than private practices? Will collaboration impact mortality or morbidity rates?

A word of caution is in order, however. The ideas assembled in this book are based on value preferences that do not lend themselves to scientific measurement but, rather, to ethical inquiry. The authors assume that comprehensive assessment is a good thing—and that comprehensive treatment or intervention is even better. There needs to be no scientific investigation with regard to the merit of collaborating; its value is clear. There may be ethical conflicts that will arise in the course of collaboration: a nurse may question the medical advice of a physician; a lawyer and a social worker may disagree about what is in the best interest of the client. These types of issues pose serious problems for professionals, but they are problems that are largely ethical in origin and which must be analyzed ethically. Ethical analysis requires the systematic listing and prioritizing of one's values in a particular conflict situation. For example, the nurse in the aforementioned situation must balance her respect for the physician's authority against her need to protect a patient.

These two separate realms of inquiry, scientific versus ethical, have their place in research. Science can shed light on the reality of a situation, yet how that reality is valued is a matter of preference. Professions must come to grips with their values in guiding practitioners' actions. The multidisciplinary approach being promoted here represents more than a technical methodology. It represents an ethical commitment.

POLICY IMPLICATIONS

One of the issues that this book indirectly addresses is whether or not increased governmental regulation is avoidable if professionals take greater responsibility for controlling their own behaviors. The policy implications of the multidisciplinary approach are not so much a matter of what policies can be expected if the approach were institutionalized as of what policies might be avoided if professionals were to take greater responsibility for regulating themselves.

It is hard to predict the implications of a multidisciplinary plan for policy development, since we are in such a state of flux regarding the prospects for legislative approval of a national health plan. Given the history of health services delivery in this country, one can expect that the system will remain fragmented (regardless of any congressional policy developments), that there still will be a role for the private insurers, and that there will continue to be both public and private tiers to the service delivery system. Basically, nothing will change if a new national health care system is set in place, except that the 12 percent of the population which currently is uninsured will receive coverage, and we will all have fewer benefits.

Government steps in when the purse strings need to be tightened or when the general welfare and health of the people need to be protected. Professions still have much discretion over the way in which their work is organized and direct services are delivered. If professionals do not make themselves accountable for ensuring that service recipients' needs are met, the government will institute additional constraints upon professional activities.

For now the choice is still ours. Professionals can try to create policy from the ground up or risk further regulation. Private independent practice is not necessarily inefficient. In fact, it is imaginable that the additional overhead involved in managing a health maintenance organization inflates, rather than controls, costs. It is also possible that entrepreneurs can take advantage of economies of scale by forming purchasing collectives (Nathanson 1993).

The precepts outlined in this book are designed to help practitioners assume greater control over their work. They represent prudent business strategy as well as solid professional activity. Policies can reinforce competent professionalism. Yet they cannot motivate professionals to do their jobs well.

OVERCOMING OBSTACLES TO
A MULTIDISCIPLINARY APPROACH

The authors describe some obstacles to the informal coordination of services and methods of overcoming these impediments. Similarly, one can foresee many potential obstacles to the formal institutionalization of a multidisciplinary approach.

The formal institutionalization of a multidisciplinary approach requires the support of professional associations and schools of higher education. It is up to umbrella organizations, such as the Association for Gerontology in Higher Education (AGHE), the Gerontological Society of America (GSA), and the American Society on Aging (ASA), to use their influence to promote collaboration among the different professional groups through the development of practice standards and training programs.

The formal institutionalization of a multidisciplinary approach can be facilitated through the efforts of consumer groups, such as the American Association for Retired Persons (AARP). Popular demand can be a forceful ally in the promotion of a cause.

The concept of a multidisciplinary approach to serving the older adults is on the verge of reaching the crest of a wave. This book may provide some new insight into the promotion of collaboration. Collaboration, however, as pointed out earlier, is not a new concept. It simply is coming around again. The authors would like to see professionals take an active, rather than reactive, stance in organizing their work—in the interest of the older adults they serve and the many fields of expertise they represent.

REFERENCE

Nathanson, R. (1993). Note from buying groups lower property insurance, by Douglas Feiden, 18. *Crain's New York Business,* 12 July.

CONCLUSION

In this book the authors have presented a framework for the integration of community services to the elderly. The approach derives from long-standing principles of interdisciplinary collaboration. The novelty of what is presented in these pages relates to the context of the application of these principles. Traditionally, collaboration has been a hallmark of professional behavior in organizational settings. The ideas elaborated in this book ask professionals to adapt principles of organizational collaboration to the less formal community practice setting. In order for this approach to be implemented, professionals must incorporate collaboration as a formal aspect of their professional function. Paradoxically, the institutionalization of this "role relationship" might better ensure the autonomy of the independent community practitioner.

The concept of role relationship is critical to an understanding of the importance of multidisciplinary collaboration. According to role theory, each professional position is assigned certain tasks, which define the scope of the professional service responsibility. The role relationship refers to the nature of the interaction among the various position holders (Nathanson 1984, 61). Professions are generally clear about what distinguishes their role from others, yet relationships among professions have not been scrutinized as closely by most professional groups. Where attention has been focused on the subject, it primarily has been oriented to the behaviors of professionals within the closed system of a hospital or agency setting. The approach presented here asks professionals not only to transcend traditional methods of role functioning in adapting methodologies to the special needs of older adults; it also asks that professionals relate to professionals from other disciplines in uncustomary ways.

Quality assurance and cost containment are the principal objectives in strategies designed to achieve health care reform. During the 1990s a health reform plan emphasized universal coverage and increased competition among insurance companies in promoting these objectives. The plan did little to address the fragmentation in the regulation and delivery of health services which is at the root of problems in the cost and quality of care. It is our belief that, despite prophecies of radical improvement in the system of health services' delivery, reform measures will continue for some time to focus on cost containment as

193

the principal target of adjustment. Managed care looms larger on the horizon, despite the politicians' assurances of the preservation of the independent practitioner model as a "consumer choice."

If professional groups want to preserve their autonomy and have anything to say about the future of health care reform, they must combine forces and establish a multidisciplinary lobby. Medicine needs the other professions in promoting an organizational approach that reflects traditional professional standards of quality. State and national professional associations are going to have to communicate with one another in establishing a consensus regarding the nature of reform. Otherwise, business factors will continue to take precedence in planning, and professional interests will be subordinated to those that are purely financial.

Reform efforts must simultaneously take place on the level of practice. This book offers one approach to reorganization which is, fundamentally, ideological. The authors believe that institutional change in service delivery can best be effected through the reassertion of traditional professional values of caring and healing. We believe that concepts of caring must be adapted to fit the complexity of today's society. People have multiple needs. Care must address the range and interplay of these needs. Caring for the elderly requires a blend of special technique and general knowledge. The specialist who sees him- or herself as a healer of one part of the patient's anatomy has no place in the community of elder practice. The elder practitioner must not only transcend norms of specialization within his or her own discipline but also must be attuned to the range of other needs impacting the client or patient's condition and be prepared to work cooperatively with practitioners from other disciplines.

In the final analysis the practice methodology outlined in this book represents a statement of what the authors believe is proper and appropriate. Aging itself is a good metaphor for the ideas presented here. Growth and aging are not parts of a linear process. It is commonly said that a person moves two steps backward for every step taken forward. This is also true of institutions. The aging of the population has placed new pressure on professions to study and evaluate traditional ways of working. Similarly, cost concerns are resulting in tighter regulation of professional activities. Perhaps the ultimate resolution to these conflicting demands lies in rapprochement, not revolution. Elder practice is about consensus building, or finding the common denominator among differing interests. It is a practice methodology based on philosophical principles of professionalism. It is, after all, why we all decided upon service careers yesterday, when we were young.

REFERENCE

Nathanson, I. (1984). Patterns of adaptation of social workers to the acute care setting. Ph.D. diss., Yeshiva University.

APPENDIX

MULTIDISCIPLINARY SCREENING INSTRUMENT (MSI)

Instructions: Indicate presence, absence, and/or need for further referral after conducting a simple, minimally structured face-to-face interview.

	YES	NO	REFERRAL
APPEARANCE			
Is the client neatly and appropriately dressed?	☐	☐	☐
Is client's clothing clean?	☐	☐	☐
Is client's hair neatly combed?	☐	☐	☐
Is the person clean?	☐	☐	☐
Does the client make eye contact?	☐	☐	☐
When he or she interacts with the interviewer, does the client make involuntary movements?	☐	☐	☐
AFFECT			
Are the client's mood and reactions appropriate to the interview situation?	☐	☐	☐
INTELLECT			
Are there any indicators that the client's level of abstract thinking is impaired?	☐	☐	☐
MEMORY			
Short-term memory determination with questions such as:			
Did you have breakfast today?	☐	☐	☐
What did you eat?	☐	☐	☐
Long-term memory determination with questions such as:			
Do you remember your birth date?	☐	☐	☐
JUDGMENT			
Does the client understand that a problem exists?	☐	☐	☐
Does the client propose a solution?	☐	☐	☐
Does the client's suggestion demonstrate a sound grasp of the current situation?	☐	☐	☐
Is the client able to recognize that one of the solutions must be implemented?	☐	☐	☐

ORIENTATION
  Is the client able to identify the date, familiar people,
    and personal identity?   □   □   □

LEVEL OF INDEPENDENCE
  Is the person able to live independently?   □   □   □

PHYSICAL LIMITATIONS
  Is the individual's ability to move hampered in any way?   □   □   □
  Is the client's hand-grip strength sufficient for ordinary
    day-to-day activities?   □   □   □
  Does the client have impaired vision?   □   □   □
  Does the client have any apparent hearing loss?   □   □   □

Associations That Participate in the National Consortium on Interprofessional Education and Practice

American Association of Colleges for Teacher Education
American Association for Colleges of Nursing
American Bar Association
American Counseling Association
American Medical Association
American Psychological Association
Association of Schools of Allied Health Professions
Association of American Law Schools
Association of Theological Schools
Commission on Interprofessional Education and Practice
Council on Social Work Education
Hebrew Union College
National Association of Social Workers
National Council of Churches
National Education Association

SOURCE: Michael R. Casto and Maria C. Julia,
Interprofessional care and collaborative practice
(Monterey, Calif.: Brooks/Cole, 1994), 104.

INDEX

Adamek, M. E., 93
Adelman, M., 157
Administration on Aging, 86
AIDS, 7, 28, 88
Albrecht, T., 157
Allen, Barbara, 91
Alzheimer's disease, 3, 13, 30, 52, 54–
    56, 59, 61, 88, 92
American Association for Retired
    Persons, 191
American Society on Aging, 191
Anderson-Ray, S., 83
Andrews, A., 24–25
Annie E. Casey Foundation, 34
Antonucci, T., 129–31
Association for Gerontology in Higher
    Education, 87, 89, 191
Ativan, 54
Austin, C., 125

Baltes, P. B. 163–64
Barresi, C., 122
Bauer, Harry, 167
Baylor University, 33–34
Beal, D. P., 89
Bill of Rights, 72
Bloom, M., 33
Blue Cross and Blue Shield, 133
Brewer, E., 87, 89
Broderick, A., 122
Brody, J. A., 10
Brown, D., 174
Butler, R., 157, 60

Cadieux, R.J., 160, 162
Caine, E. D., 49, 53
Campbell, A., 130
Cantor, M. H., 125, 129–30
Casto, R. M., 25–27, 33–34
Catastrophic Health Care Act, 17
Cath, S., 120
Chaim, Hofetz, 81
Chandy, J., 100
Chaplin, Charlie, 188
Chown, S. M., 154
Clinton, William Jefferson, 2
Clozapine, 59
Cohler, B., 125
Cole, Thomas, 80
Cole, T. R., 90
Coward, R. T., 125
Cox, C., 10, 18, 24
Cox, E. O., 135–36
Cuellar, J. B., 122
Cummings, S. R., 45

Dana, B., 174
Davies, J., 29
Declaration of Independence, 72
Dunkel, R. E., 13
Dychtwald, K., 133

Eaton, Anne, 133
Education and Human Services
    Consortium, 33
Elavil, 53
Ellor, J. W., 83
The Encyclopedia of Social Work, 24
English, J., 100

Estes, C. L., 9, 19, 33, 38
Euster, G. L., 81, 87

Farkas, K., 13, 41, 93
Federal Register, 32
Field, P., 129
Fineman, N., 99
Focal Point, 108
Ford Foundation, 34
Fordham University's Third Age Center, 80, 85
Foster, Z., 174
Fowler, J., 68
Fox, R., 174
Frank, L., 35
Freedman, R., 68
Freidson, E., 1
Fries, J., 9

Gelfand, D., 122
Germain, C. B., 117
Gerontological Society of America, 24, 191
Gibson, R. C., 48–49
Ginsberg, L., 8–9
Glover, S., 81
Gold, N., 180
Goodfellow, M., 122, 132
Grant, L. A., 7–8, 11–12
Green, Jacob, 167
Green, Mildred, 167
Greene, R. R., 155
Gurian, B., 130
Gutheil, I., 8, 10

Harel, Z., 127
Harkins, E. B., 156
Harrington, Barbara, 168
Harrington, C., 9, 19, 33, 38
Harrington, Mabel, 168
Harrington, Tim, 168
Harris, P. R., 102

Harvard Health Letter, 70
Haven, C., 129
Health Care Financing Administration, 179
Hendricks, D. C., 17, 23, 42–44, 55, 119
Hendricks, J., 17, 23, 42–44, 55, 119
Hepworth, D. H., 116, 117
Hirayama, H., 134
Hommel, M., 105
Hooyman, N. R., 7–9, 11, 13, 15, 16, 38–45, 48, 79, 82–83
Hornbrook, M. C., 45

ICD-9-CM manual, 17
Institute of Medicine, 105
Interdisciplinary Health Care Team, 33

Jette, C. B., 125
Johnson, C. L., 7–8, 11–12
Johnson, Lyndon Baines, 1
Johnson, R. J., 10, 38
Johnson, S., 93
Joint Commission on Accreditation of Health Organizations, 179
Journal of Interprofessional Care, 33
Journal of Religion and Aging, 87
Journal of Religious Gerontology, 87
Journey of Life (paintings), 80
Julia, M. C., 25–27, 33–34
Jung, Carl, 90

Kahn, A. J., 132
Kahn, R., 175
Kahn, R. L., 129–30
Kaplan, M. S., 93
Kastenbaum, R., 165
Katz, D., 175
Katz, S., 10
Kennedy, John Fitzgerald, 1
Kerr, P., 69
Kim, S. S., 100
King, D. A., 49, 53

Kingson, N. R., 17
Kiyak, A. H., 7–9, 11, 13, 15–16, 38–45, 48, 79, 82–83
Knight, B., 129
Korsakov's psychosis, 60–61
Kramer, M., 33
Krause, N., 124
Kreps, G. L., 169
Kropf, N. P., 129

Lamy, P. P., 56
Langer, N., 106
Laux, L., 105
Leininger, M., 100
Lewis, M., 157, 160
Lewis, M. A., 80, 84–87
Libby, J., 70
Life Enrichment Services, 133
Listan, M., 174
Litwak, E., 131
locus of control theory, 179
Longres, J., 135
Lowenthal, M. F., 129
Lyness, J. M., 49, 53

Macera, C. A., 32
Mailbach, E. W., 169
MAO inhibitors, 53
Marine Nursing Home, 46
Markides, K. S., 122, 124
Mayer, M. J., 125
Mayewski, R., 45
Meals of Wheels, 68, 85, 126
Medicaid, 1–2, 11, 14–21, 31, 33, 66, 69, 85, 104, 141, 143, 149
Medicare, 1–2, 11, 15–17, 19–21, 31, 33, 69, 85, 104, 133, 141, 143, 179
Medicare Prospective Payment Plan, 17
Merrill, J. M., 105
Mindel, C., 122
Moberg, D. O., 79, 89
Modern Times (film), 188

Moody, H. R., 90
Moran, R. T., 102
Morgan, R., 80, 81, 84
Morse, J. M., 100
Mullaney, J., 174
Multidisciplinary Screening Instrument, 2, 4, 184
Multi-Infarct Dementia, 55
Mutran, E., 125

Nardil, 53
Nathanson, I., 75, 175, 193
Nathanson, R., 191
National Association of Areawide Agencies on Aging, 86
National Association of State Units on Aging, 86
National Center for Health Statistics, 11, 37–38
National Conference of Catholic Bishops, 85
National Consortium on Interprofessional Education and Practice, 33
National Health Interview Study, 9
National Interfaith Coalition, 83
National Long-Term Care Channeling Demonstration Program, 18
National Survey of Black Americans, 81
Nebraska State Bar Association v. Walsh, 105
Neparstek, A., 128
Neugarten, R. L., 83
Nevitt, M. C. 45
Newcomer, R. J., 9, 19, 33, 38
Nopramin, 53
No Wrinkles on the Soul, 83

Ohio Commission on Interprofessional Education and Practice, 34
Older Americans Act, 14
Omnibus Reconciliation Act, 29

On Lok program, 18
O'Rourke, K., 75
Osgood, N., 156

Pamelor, 53
Parkinson's disease, 45, 57, 59
Parnate, 53
Payne, B., 87, 89
Peters, J. E., 75
Professional Review Organization, 179
Prozac, 53–54

Raschko, R., 129
Regan, J. J., 104
Reinhart, R., 129
Reitzes, D. C., 125
Retired Senior Volunteer Program, 132
Robinson, P. K., 75
Rosenfeld, J., 116

Scheidt, R. A., 122
Schneider, E. L., 10
Schneider, L., 129
Shulman, L., 174
Silverstone, B., 111
Sinkler-Parker, C., 81
Slocum, H., 100
Smith, J. M., 81
Social Security, 17, 64, 66–67, 70, 104, 143, 148, 153
Social Security Act, 11, 14, 17
Social Security Administration, 69
Sol, Jacqueline, 30, 31
Sol, John, 30, 31
Solomon, K., 13
St. Christopher's Home, 84–85
State Units on Aging, 86
Stoller, E., 48–49
Supplemental Security Income, 14, 67, 70, 104

Taylor, R. J., 79, 81, 82

Tinetti, M. E., 45
Tirrito, T., 16, 18, 81, 87
Tobin, S. S., 79, 82–83
Toframil, 53
Toner, J. A., 14
Travis, J., 55
Turner, F., 6, 84
Tuzman, L., 174

University of Washington at Seattle, 34
U. S. Bureau of the Census, 41, 80
U. S. Health Care Financing Administration, 32

Valium, 54
Verbrugge, L. M., 9, 10
Virginia Department for the Aging, 129
Virginia Power, 129

WanderPolo, M., 68
War on Poverty, 1
Wasser, E., 112
Weeks, J., 122
Wells Fargo, 133
Wentowski, G. J., 131
Wernicke's encephalopathy, 60
Wiemann, J. M., 101
Williams, F. T., 45
Wimpfheimer, R., 33
Winnett, R. L., 125
W. K. Kellogg Foundation, 34
Wolinsky, F. D., 10, 38
World Health Organization, 8, 39
Wylie, M., 125

Xanax, 54

Yates, B., 70

Zarit, S. H., 158
Zoloft, 53